# Which Natural Therapies Should You Try?

A simple guide to natural treatments

Dr. Shaun Holt & Emma Dalton

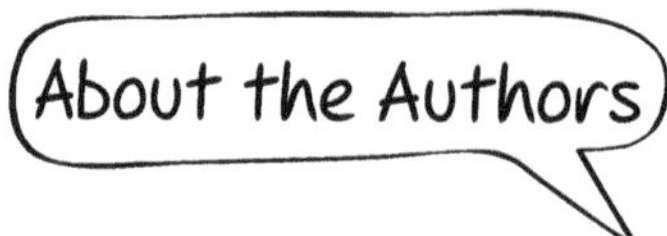


**Dr. Shaun Holt** is the founder of two clinical trial organisations and Research Review, a company that produces regular reviews of the medical literature for health professionals. Shaun holds Pharmacy and Medicine degrees, has been the Principal Investigator in over 50 clinical trials and has over 160 publications in medical literature. He is the Science Director of HoneyLab, an Advisor to the Asthma and Respiratory Foundation and Natural Products New Zealand, a regular contributor on TV One's Breakfast program and national radio shows. Shaun lectures at the Victoria University of Wellington, is on the editorial board of two complementary medicine journals and has previously written six books on health topics. In 2015 he was one of three finalists for the New Zealander of the Year Awards - Innovator of the Year. More information can be found at http://flavors.me/shaunholt

**Emma Dalton** hated english at school. This didn't stop her from jumping at the chance to write a book with her uncle Shaun though. She loves science and is planning on studying biological science at university. In her free time she likes to sail with her dad, go out for coffee with her mum and travel the world with her brother.

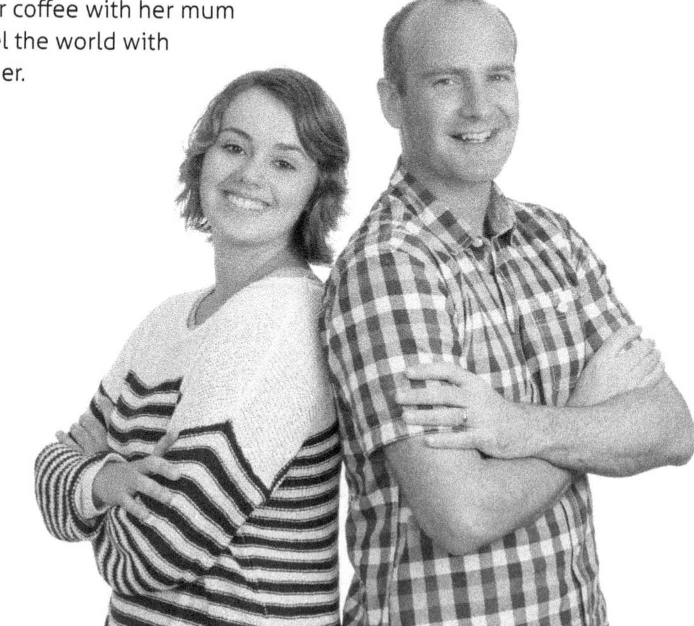

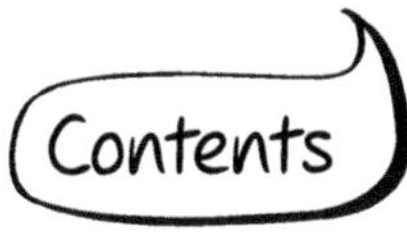



| | | |
|---|---|---|
| **01** | How we know which natural therapies can help? | **1** |
| **02** | Weight loss and exercise | **9** |
| **03** | Pain | **17** |
| **04** | Breathing | **25** |
| **05** | Diabetes | **33** |
| **06** | Heart and blood | **41** |
| **07** | Stomach and bowels | **53** |
| **08** | Brain and nervous system | **61** |
| **09** | Mental health | **71** |
| **10** | Bones and joints | **81** |
| **11** | Cancer prevention | **89** |
| **12** | Women's health | **95** |
| **13** | Children's health | **101** |
| **14** | Elderly health | **107** |
| **15** | Other health issues | **113** |
| **16** | Staying safe with natural therapies | **121** |
| Index 1 - Conditions | | **125** |
| Index 2 - Therapies | | **131** |

First published December, 2016, Tauranga, New Zealand



The information contained in this book is intended to provide accurate and helpful health information for the general public. It is made available on the understanding that the authors and publisher are not engaged in rendering medical, health, psychological, or any other kind of personal professional services in this book. The information should not be considered complete and does not cover all diseases, ailments, physical conditions or their treatment. It should not be used in place of a visit to a medical, health or other competent professional, who should be consulted before adopting any of the suggestions contained within.

The information about health products contained in this book is general in nature. It does not cover all possible uses, actions, precautions, side effects, or interactions of the products mentioned. The information is not intended as medical advice for individual problems or for making an evaluation as to the risks and benefits of taking a particular health product.

The authors and publisher specifically disclaim all responsibility for any liability, loss or risk, personal or otherwise, which is incurred as a consequence, directly or indirectly, of the use and application of any of the material in this book.

ISBN: 978-0-9876617-4-6

CHAPTER 01

# How do we know which natural therapies can help?

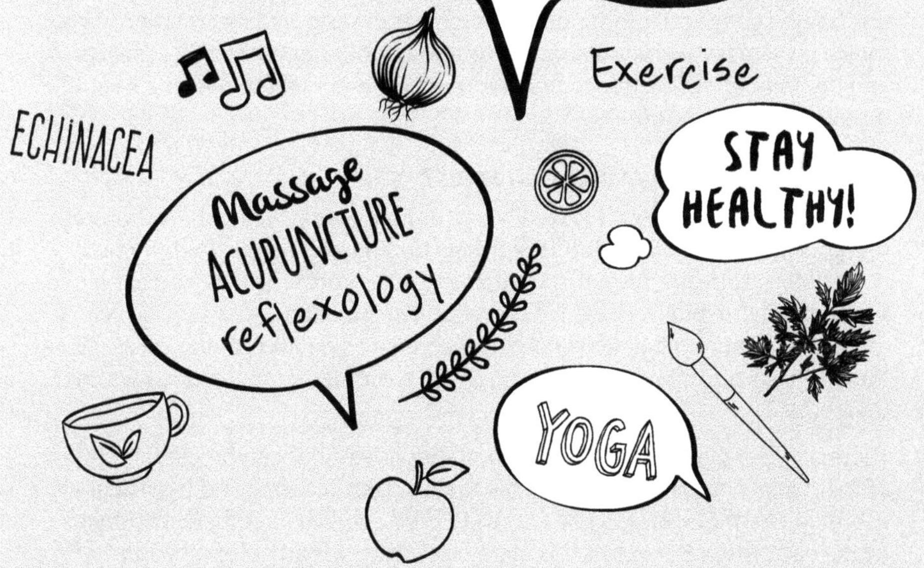

## Do we need another book on this?

There are lots of ways to get information on natural therapies. In fact it's hard to avoid it. We see stories on natural therapies in newspapers, magazines and on the TV all the time. There are also hundreds of books on the subject. So why did we write yet another book? The reason is simple in our humble opinion, it has not been done well before.

The aim of this book is to give an overview of those natural therapies with the most scientific evidence that can help with your health. It is deliberately short, but ambitious in that we try to cover the best natural therapies for a wide range of health issues. There is no way that we could go into great detail about the several hundred natural therapies that we cover, so just the briefest of overviews is given. This is important to understand: the aim of this book is simply to point you in the right direction. Please do not make any decisions based on the information in this book. Instead, think of it as a sieve whereby we have presented only the best natural therapies (from the thousands available) so that you can quickly see which ones you can look into in more detail.

In the opening chapter we will look briefly at what natural therapies actually are, how to get good information on them (and avoid bad information). Why they are increasingly popular and a little bit about good and bad research and the strength of evidence that supports (or doesn't) the use of a natural therapy for a condition.

## What actually are natural therapies?

Before going any further it is well worth defining what we mean by natural therapies, as it can mean different things to different people. A definition that I like is '*self-care system of natural therapies concerned with building and restoring health and wellness via prevention and healthy lifestyles.*' As well as natural treatments it also includes diet, exercise, naturopathy, massage therapy, relaxation techniques, acupuncture, aromatherapy and many other therapies.

There are literally thousands of natural therapies, so it can be useful to think of them in groups. There are several official classifications and a particularly useful one is that which is used by the *Encyclopaedia of Complementary Medicine* (Carlton Books). In this large book they put all natural health therapies into one of seven classifications:

| GROUP | COMMON EXAMPLES |
|---|---|
| **Natural Healing** | Colour therapy, homeopathy, iridology |
| **Herbal Medicine** | Herbs, flower essences |
| **Nutrition and Diet** | Diets, naturopathic medicine |
| **Mobility and Posture** | Chiropractic, osteopathy, yoga, Alexander technique |
| **The Mind** | Hypnotherapy, meditation, music therapy |
| **Massage and Touch** | Massage, aromatherapy, reflexology |
| **Eastern Therapies** | Acupuncture, acupressure, Chinese herbal medicine |

It is said that unlike standard medical care, natural therapies try to not only treat the specific problem, but also the whole body, the mind and the spirit i.e. the holistic approach. This is however a little harsh on doctors who do try to help with both physical and mental health issues, and are usually strong advocates for leading a healthy lifestyle with plenty of exercise and good nutrition.

However, it is true that mind-body interactions are not well understood by conventional scientific methods and we have little understanding on how therapies like hypnosis or music therapy work. But they certainly do work and it is worth remembering that as long as a therapy works (and is safe) we do not necessarily have to understand how it works.

## Getting good information

As we have already said, there are lots of stories in the media about natural products and therapies, so many in fact that it's hard to avoid them. The problem is, sadly, they cannot always be trusted to give good advice. Almost always the stories are written or presented by journalists who are not trained scientists. Often, they will simply take the contents of a press release, tweak it slightly and put it out as a story, usually with an attention-grabbing headline. The people putting out the press releases on which these stories are made can often have an agenda themselves, often to sell more products. The media often gets it wrong when they promote natural therapies based on little or no research. They also get it wrong when they write scare stories about natural therapies. One of the worst examples seen recently was headlines all round the world saying that omega-3 fish oil supplements can cause a nasty form of lethal prostate cancer. The actual research that this was based on did not prove any such thing.

As well as media stories in the newspapers, magazines and on TV, the other main source of information these days is of course the internet. More and more, people are looking to gather health information in order to take control of health decisions and therapies they should use. Unfortunately the situation here can be worse than in other forms of media. Some of the websites on natural therapies give terrible, misleading, expensive and often dangerous advice. The problem is that it is hard for people who are not doctors or trained scientists to work out whether the advice is bad. On the surface it often looks good, the people appear well qualified and there seems to be lots of scientific studies that support what they are saying. These websites can easily fool non-scientists with what we call 'pseudoscience' - it looks scientific with the medical jargon that is being used, but in reality it is no such thing.

On a positive note, there is one website which gives excellent advice on natural therapies and that is the Mayo Clinic website, which is free to access - http://www.mayoclinic.org

The only good way to get solid information on which natural therapies are effective and safe is to read the actual studies published in the medical journals. Unfortunately, this is almost impossible for a non-scientist to do as they are written in scientific jargon. It would also cost you a fortune, for example it can cost over US$30 just to have access to one paper for 24 hours! This is why we have written this book, summarising what the medical journals are saying, in easy to understand language.

## Why are natural therapies so popular?

Another reason for writing this book is that natural therapies are gaining in popularity. People want to take control of health decisions and health information is one of the most common things that people search for on the internet. Natural therapies appeal to a lot of people as they do not need to see a doctor to get a prescription for them, they can buy the product or see a practitioner themselves and decide for themselves whether the therapy works for them and whether to carry on with it or not.

Natural therapies are particularly popular where traditional medicine often fails to achieve good results, such as with back pain, preventing the common cold and conditions such as fibromyalgia.

There are many times when it would be foolish to use a natural therapy rather than a doctor-prescribed medication, examples being broken limbs, people who need treatments for cancer or an infection that needs antibiotics. However, even in these situations, there may be a role for natural therapies in addition to the doctor-prescribed treatment, for example, to combat some of the side effects. A good example of this would be when people who are having chemotherapy for cancer take ginger to reduce the nausea that is almost always caused by these powerful medicines. Another example is when people take probiotic supplements to prevent the diarrhoea that often occurs when we take antibiotics to treat infections.

This is most certainly not a book that will be critical of standard medicines and treatments that we get from doctors and hospitals. Modern conventional treatments are now usually safe and are often very effective. Simple painkillers and antibiotics can dramatically improve the symptoms of many illnesses and there are highly complex and effective treatments available for serious illnesses such as cancer. Yes, some of these treatments can have unpleasant side effects, but the benefits almost always outweigh the negative aspects. Medical treatments are improving all the time but there are still many ways that natural therapies can assist your health and most of this book discusses these therapies and the medical conditions that they can help with.

## A little bit of information about medical research

Huge textbooks have been written about the best ways to undertake research and whole sections of libraries are devoted to books on how to statistically analyse data. Don't worry, that certainly won't be happening in this book. The basic principles of medical research are actually pretty straightforward and after reading the next few paragraphs you will be in a better position to make your own informed decisions on the merits of medical research studies.

The first clue as to whether medical research is good or not, is to look at where the research was published. There are around 10,000 medical journals and they are ranked in order of importance, the so-called 'Impact Factor'. It's very similar to the football league table for the English Premier League. Near the top of the list are the famous medical journals such as the *British Medical Journal, The Lancet and the New England Journal of Medicine*. In general, the best studies appear in the better journals. Researchers want to publish their work in the best place that they can and the best journals generally only publish the best research.

The better journals have a system in place known as 'peer review' and it involves the research paper being sent to several experts who look at the paper in great detail, they make comments on the paper and give their opinion as to whether the paper should be published. Usually they will either reject the paper, or suggest that it is published but with a few changes. The whole process is done anonymously in order to prevent the experts from deliberately stopping the publication of their academic rivals! Again, although not fool proof, a paper published in a peer-reviewed journal is likely to be of a high standard.

There are many ways of undertaking medical research, but the 'gold standard' or best way has a fancy name of 'a randomised controlled trial' (or RCT). In a typical RCT the participants (or subjects) are randomly chosen to either get the treatment that is being tested or a control, commonly called a placebo (or fake treatment). The two groups are then followed over a fixed period of time and at the end the results of the two groups are compared. Ideally, this comparison is undertaken in a 'blind' manner, where the subjects do not know who has received the active treatment and who have received the placebo. If possible, the study is also 'double-blind', this means that not only do the subjects not know who is receiving the treatment, but the researchers undertaking the study and recording the data do not know either. Although a RCT is a simple method for undertaking clinical research, as you can see, it is actually very powerful.

The final idea about medical research is what we call 'levels of evidence'. We are all pretty familiar with the levels of evidence in the legal setting: if I shoot someone in front of 100 witnesses, their testimony would be stronger evidence of me committing the crime compared to only having my fingerprints found at the crime scene. Most of us are also pretty comfortable with the process of giving more weight to strong evidence and less weight to weaker evidence. It is no different with medical research - when deciding if a therapy is likely to work or not, we look at all the evidence available and give more weight to the better quality evidence before making a decision.

In this book, all that work has been done for you! Please remember though, just like in a court of law, sometimes it is not possible to make a definite decision even after looking at the evidence. There may be contradictory evidence, or there may not be much evidence to look at in the first place. Also, for a variety of reasons, not all therapies work for everyone - we are all different and react differently. That is why you will see a lot of 'weasel words' in the book such as 'may', 'can', 'likely', just to remind you that nothing is guaranteed. The best we can say for a natural therapy is that there has been a lot of research and it looks like for most people, that it is safe and effective.

It is also worth pointing out that in some ways the medical research of natural therapies can be a bit different to medical research of pharmaceutical medicines. For a start, there is nowhere near as much research done on natural therapies as is done on pharmaceutical medicines and the reason is ..... money. The pharmaceutical industry spends more than US$60 billion each year on the research and development of new medications. Compared to that, the amount that is spent on natural health research is only a fraction and so there are far fewer studies and less research available to make decisions on.

The main reason for this difference is the lack of patent protection for many natural health therapies and treatments. A patent is defined as *'a set of exclusive rights granted by a state to the inventor for a fixed period of time'* and the period of time is usually around 17 years. Pharmaceutical companies can patent the medicines that they invent as they are new, but it's very hard to do this with natural therapies that have already been around for hundreds of years.

One final thought before you get into the main part of this book. You will see lots of different types of therapies in this book.....there are arty ones like music therapy, more spiritual ones like meditation, some physical ones like massage along with diets that can help and pills you can take. One of the great things about natural therapies is that there is usually something for everyone. More than that, there may well be several therapies that you might want to try, it does not have to be limited to just one. You may decide that natural therapies are not for you, but at least you'll have made a decision based on good information. As we've already said, nothing works for everyone and almost certainly there will be some trial-and-error before you find one (or more) therapies that work for you. Above all, we hope that you find this book to be a useful overview of natural therapies, so you know a bit about a lot of them and have an idea which ones you want to learn more about or try. Above all, the main thing is to *stay healthy!*

CHAPTER 02

# Weight loss and exercise

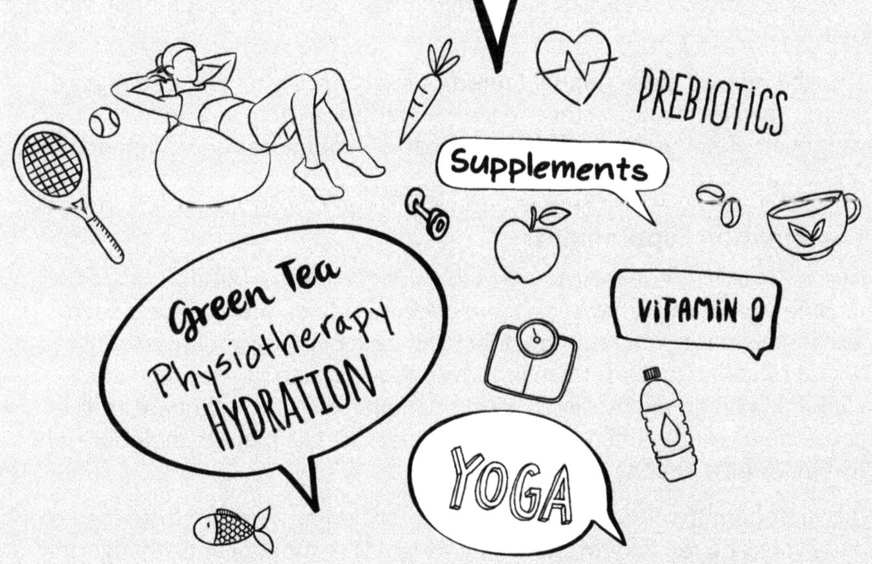

Of course you know how important exercise is in order to maintain a healthy weight. Exercise increases your energy levels, boosts your focus and problem-solving abilities and can be a great way to relax. It can protect you from many diseases and health problems; heart disease, strokes, type 2 diabetes and arthritis to name just a few. It has been estimated that being overweight by as little as 10 kg means your body contains an extra 8,000 km of blood vessels that your heart has to pump blood through. Your heart won't be the only one thanking you for staying fit; being fit means you are more relaxed, less stressed which makes you less irritable. This can improve relationships in all the important parts of your life.

Yet despite all this, over ⅓ of adults are overweight and more than 80% do not meet the recommended guidelines for the amount of exercise you should do each week - the current recommendations are around 150 minutes a week of moderate aerobic activity or 75 minutes a week of vigorous aerobic activity. Sticking to a workout routine or diet can be tough; most people give up within a few months. It can be hard to see immediate benefits and this can make the exercise seem pointless. Injuries can also stop people from working out.

This chapter will cover natural therapies to enhance your exercise regime so you can see results faster and supplements that help you keep extra weight off. Helping you recover from post-workout aches and common sports injuries are also covered.

## Combination Supplements

Getting your heart beating faster is the aim of exercise, but does increasing it using supplements have the same effect? Many natural products such as caffeine make your heart beat fast and can speed up your metabolism. A study showed that after two months people who took a supplement containing green tea extract, tyrosine, caffeine, calcium carbonate and capsaicin as well as following a healthy diet lost 1kg more than people who just followed a healthy diet.

It is important to follow a healthy lifestyle including a healthy balanced diet and exercising regularly while taking weight loss supplements, though they help, they cannot do all the work for you. However, this supplement combo (or similar variations of it) can provide a boost to speed the process a little.

## Calcium

Calcium is important for keeping your bones strong as you grow older, but it has another interesting use. Calcium supplements may help women reduce their weight gain. After the onset of menopause, many women continue to gain weight until they are in their 60s. A massive study of 10,000 women showed that those who regularly took a calcium supplement gained 2kg less than women who did not.

You probably know that one of the best sources of calcium is from dairy products. However many dairy products contain lots of calories, so eating too much might not be a good idea for losing weight! Choosing low-fat unsweetened options are one possibility. Eating lots of leafy green vegetables and legumes like beans and lentils can add extra calcium to your diet, while keeping your meals healthy. Alternatively calcium supplements might be the way to go for the easiest way to increase your calcium levels. There are many forms of calcium and some of the cheaper forms like Calcium Carbonate (chalk/dolomite) are not very well absorbed.

## Prebiotics

Prebiotics are the fuel that the good bacteria in your body use to grow. The bacteria that help you break down the nutrients in your food use prebiotics as a fertiliser. Making sure you get enough prebiotics is important to keep the bacteria in your digestive system working properly. Increasing your intake of prebiotics might help you maintain a healthy body weight, especially during adolescence. A yearlong study of children in their first stages of puberty showed that those who took a prebiotic supplement had less body fat and had a lower BMI.

*BMI stands for Body Mass Index. It gives you an idea of whether you're underweight, overweight or an ideal weight for your height. There are lots of calculators online that will work out your BMI for you. There are 4 groups that your BMI result can place you in: underweight less than 18.5, normal weight between 18.5 and 24.9, overweight between 25 and 29.9, obese = 30 or greater.*

You get the most prebiotics out of raw food. Raw onion has double the amount of prebiotics in it than the same weight of cooked onion. While raw onion might not sound too appealing, it can taste great in salads, burgers, sandwiches and salsa dressings. Bananas and asparagus also contain lots of prebiotics, as does whole-wheat flour.

## Green Tea

Made from the same plant as other types of tea, green tea leaves simply have not been dried as much as regular tea. This dates back to the reign of Emperor Shennong in China and legend has it that he experimented with the effects of different plants on the human body and in 2,473 BC was the first to discover tea as an antidote. Drinking green tea can help you lose weight by enhancing the effects of exercise. A three month study showed that people who drank a cup of green tea every day lost more weight and more fat than people who had other hot beverages.

Tea Bags are available at supermarkets, or you can buy green tea leaves to brew yourself at home.

### Zinc

Found in deodorants, shampoos, batteries and paints, zinc is more common than most people think. Its name comes from the German word *zinke* which means tooth-like. This is because zinc crystals can form sharp pointy shapes, like a predator's teeth. Not having enough zinc in your body can noticeably reduce your exercise performance. Zinc is important in many parts of your body you use when you work out, including your heart, lungs and blood.

Oysters are a food you may want to try to increase your zinc levels, but if that doesn't appeal, meat, beans, nuts and grains are all other great sources of it. Supplements are also available and zinc is usually an ingredient in most multivitamins.

### L-arginine

Proteins are large molecules that carry out all sorts of important jobs in your cells. They are made of smaller building blocks called amino acids. One of these amino acids is L-arginine which is essential for helping your body heal, especially after burns, infections and cuts. Not many people know that it can also improve your ability to exercise. Decreased heart rates and other signs of improved fitness in a study of people taking L-arginine showed that having plenty of it makes you cope better with exercise. It can also be helpful for people with mild heart conditions, but should be avoided by people with more serious conditions or anyone recovering from a heart attack.

Your body makes its own L-arginine in your kidneys and liver. Poultry is a great food source, turkey and chicken both have high levels of L-arginine in them. It can also be used as an excuse to tuck into a chocolate bar, as cocoa is another food containing lots of this amino acid.

### L-ornithine

This is another amino acid. Its job is to turn toxic ammonia released by your cells into a substance that your kidneys can get rid of more easily. There are also studies that have found that increasing your L-ornithine levels can give you more energy and help you recover from exercise quicker. For reasons that we do not understand, this effect was more evident in women than men. L-ornithine can make your energy consumption more efficient, therefore improving your performance when exercising.

L-ornithine is not available from food sources in very high levels. A nutritional supplement is recommended if you want to see these benefits to your exercise program.

## Hydration

In the 1960s a Florida college football team assistant coach saw that his players were suffering from playing in the hot, humid conditions. Together with a group of scientists he devised the world's first ever sports drink, made of water, sugar, salt, potassium and lemon juice. The team began winning all of their games and went on to claim first place in their league; a first for their school. Sports drinks aim to replace electrolytes that you lose through sweat keeping you more hydrated for longer.

> *Electrolytes are the minerals that your body uses to carry an electrical charge to the cells and are sweated out or used during exercise. They include sodium, potassium, calcium, magnesium, chloride.*

A study of teenagers showed that drinking sports drinks keeps your body temperature lower than drinking water does. It may seem silly but it is possible to hydrate yourself too much. Drinking too much water, too fast, can cause a rare condition called water intoxication, which can be deadly. If you are well hydrated your urine will be clear or light yellow.

Sports drinks are available in the soft drink aisle at your local supermarket and there are recipes on the internet that show you how to make your own.

## Fish Oil

Fish like salmon or tuna are often eaten for their fish oil content, but they do not actually make the omega-3 oil themselves. Over their lifetime they accumulate it in their body from the microalgae they, or even their prey, has eaten.

If you are exercising to reduce your risk of heart disease or to help lose weight, fish oil supplements can help increase the benefits of your workouts. A study showed that taking fish oil and exercising regularly improved your heart's health more effectively than either treatment did on its own.

Experts recommend eating one serving of omega-3 fatty acids each day. A serving of fish, a tablespoon of canola oil or a handful of walnuts all meet this requirement. You can also buy fish oil supplements if you want an easy, regular way to get the recommended level - look for high levels of DHA and EPA.

## Physiotherapy

Hippocrates is thought to be the first supporter of physiotherapy. It is a rehabilitative medicine, helping people to recover after an injury has happened. Tennis elbow is a condition that is not always a result of playing tennis. It causes the outside of your elbow to swell painfully, making it difficult to move your joint. Physiotherapy may be the answer if you are suffering from tennis elbow. A study of 200 people showed that eight sessions of physiotherapy was more effective than the common '*wait-and-see*' method in the short term and stopped re-injury more than corticosteroid injections in the long term.

A trained physiotherapist can do specific elbow manipulations and other therapeutic actions to help your recovery. They may also give you exercises and equipment to use at home between appointments such as a resistance exercise band.

## Caffeine

In the western world, nine out of ten of us consume caffeine every day. It is the most widely consumed psychoactive drug. It's known for keeping you alert and awake, great for finishing late night projects or for early morning starts....or for writing books! It also may have a use to help you recover after exercise.

Two cups of brewed coffee was shown to help reduce muscle pain after people trained harder than they did before. It also delayed muscle injury and lessened the loss in muscle force. This effect was most obvious in people who did not normally drink a lot of caffeine in their everyday lives.

*As caffeine is a stimulant it can stop you sleeping. It lasts for several hours in the body and if you are sensitive to caffeine you might want to avoid it completely in the evening, and even in the afternoon.*

A hot beverage is the most common source of caffeine. Tea, coffee, and hot chocolate all contain it. If you don't want to consume two full cups of coffee after exercising, supplements are available.

### Icing a Sprain

R.I.C.E. stands for rest, ice, compression and elevation. You may know that this is how to deal with a sprained ankle joint, but how exactly do you apply each step? A study found that the best way to ice a sprain is not to continuously hold the ice against it, as your instincts might suggest.

Instead, the best thing to do is place the ice pack on the sprain for 10 minutes, take a 10 minute break, and then re-apply it for another 10 minutes. This should then be repeated every two hours. Doing this reduces the pain and swelling most effectively.

### Deep Heat

Capsaicin is the spicy part of chilli peppers. It will produce a hot sensation in any part of your body that it comes into contact with. It is a natural ingredient often used in deep heat rubs that help to relieve muscle and joint pain after exercise or injury.

*The feeling of warmth Capsaicin produces may initially increase the pain, but when applied a second or third time it will help relax your muscles and the pain should decrease.*

When you apply it, be careful to keep away from anything sensitive like your eyes, nose and ears as they will sting if they come into contact with the cream! Some people wear disposable gloves when they apply it, a sensible precaution as it can be very powerful.

Deep heat rubs are available at pharmacies, you can ask the pharmacist for the 'chilli pepper cream' and they will know what you mean.

### Honey

In the case of cuts and open wounds from exercising that need a bandage, honey might just do the trick. Humans began hunting for honey over 8,000 years ago by stealing it from wild hives. Now honey farms provide a much easier way to gather the sweet, sticky substance. As well as being delicious, honey can help speed up the healing of wounds, reduce swelling and make it less likely that a scar will form.

Bandages with honey pre-applied can be an easy, mess-free way to apply honey to your wound. Jars and tubes of honey can also be bought, but make sure you only use medical-grade (sterile) honey on open cuts. Regular honey has not been purified to the same level, so you risk infection or an allergic reaction by applying it to broken skin.

## Vitamin D

Staying out of the sun can do more than just keep your skin pale. Not getting enough vitamin D is linked with a higher risk of gaining weight and becoming overweight or obese. Increasing your vitamin D levels may also make it easier for you to lose weight. A study of 400 people found that taking vitamin D while following a healthy diet led to losing double the amount of weight compared to people who just ate a healthy diet.

Other than spending more time taking in the sunlight, the amount of vitamin D in your body can be increased by eating more of certain foods. Oily fish, cheese and egg yolks all contain vitamin D. Lots of food has vitamin D added to them, just check out the nutrition information on things like cereals and dairy products. Supplements can also be taken, look for natural vitamin D3 (cholecalciferol) and take with the largest meal of the day.

## Probiotics

Doctors have only known about probiotics and their important role in breaking down food in our intestines since the 1990s. They help you absorb nutrients from food properly and make sure you get the most out of what you eat. New research is finding that probiotics can potentially help you reach your weight loss goal as well. A three month study showed that women who took probiotic capsules daily, lost over 1.5 times the weight compared to women who didn't take them. Oddly, there was no effect on men's weight loss though.

Yakult was the first probiotic food sold back in 1935. Now many products are available and the trend for probiotics to be added to food has increased.

*Take note of the amount of probiotics in each product though, as sometimes not very much is included. The dose that you should be aiming for is 5 billion bacteria per day. Not sure how they count them though!*

You can ensure a consistent high dose of probiotics by taking a supplement. Look for a supplement where the probiotics are protected from stomach acid with acid resistant capsules or a special coating.

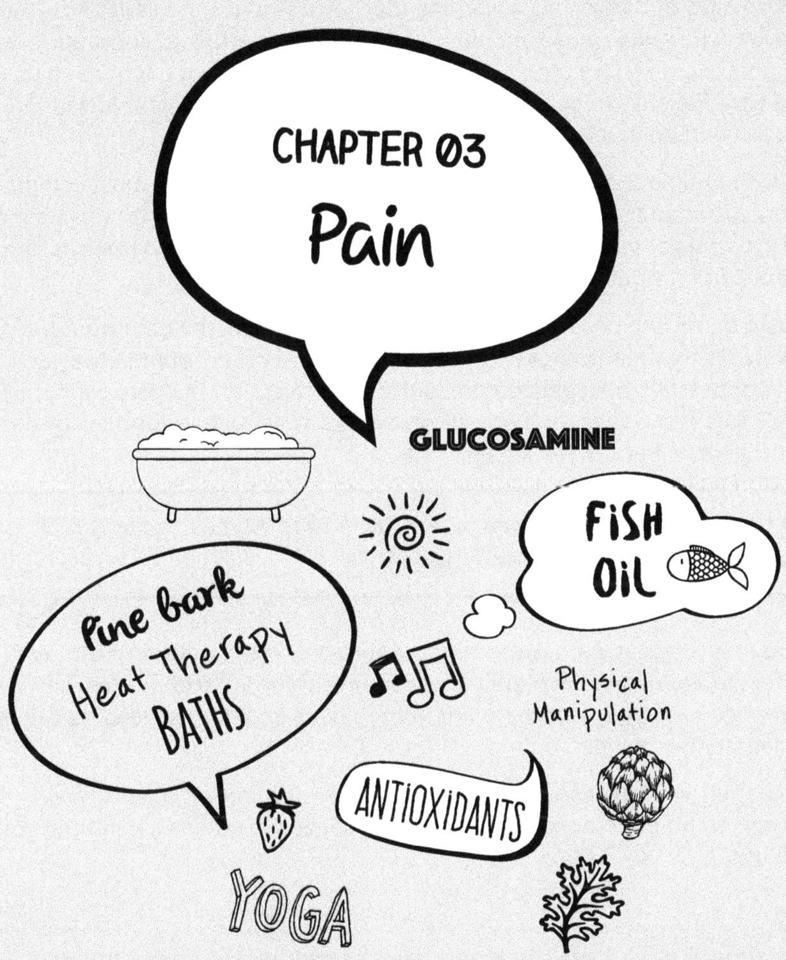
CHAPTER 03
Pain
GLUCOSAMINE
FiSH OiL
Pine bark
Heat Therapy
BATHS
Physical Manipulation
ANTIOXIDANTS
YOGA

When you get hurt, it's not actually your body that's hurting at all. It's just your brain telling you that your body hurts. Pain has evolved as a natural defence against danger. It's a warning that says '*stop doing this, it's not good for you.*' It was important back when we were getting to know our environment, when we didn't know what was poisonous or might harm us in some way. Pain has to be painful because if it wasn't, you might just ignore it and then end up in a very bad way!

Pain is the number one symptom in many illnesses and is the most common reason you would see a doctor. It helps your doctor diagnose what is wrong with you and get you on the right course of treatment. So pain really is very helpful, until it's not!

It would be nice if, once your condition was diagnosed, the pain would go away. As treatments kick in, this is normally the case, but not always. What about when pain gets out of control or a cause for the pain cannot be found? This is the case for many chronic conditions such as fibromyalgia and recurring knee, back or neck pain.

*The name fibromyalgia means pain in the bodies' fibrous tissues, which are your muscles, tendons and ligaments.*

As this may suggest, pain is the main symptom of this condition. Sufferers also feel fatigued and have difficulty sleeping. Over 50% of people will experience back pain at some point in their lives and it is the leading cause of disability worldwide.

This chapter will cover some natural remedies for different types of pain and ways to lift your mood if all the aches, pains and strains are getting you down.

## Yoga

Originating in India, Yoga combines various poses with different breathing methods and meditation. It is practiced by millions of people worldwide as a way of keeping fit and relaxing. Among many other health benefits, Yoga may also reduce any lower back pain you are experiencing. It may put you in a better mood and may mean you can take fewer painkillers.

A study of over 100 people revealed that people who attended a Yoga class a couple of times a week were more flexible and able to carry out tasks that involved them flexing their backs.

There are many different types of Yoga and you can choose the style that best suits your fitness level and personality. Hatha Yoga is gentle and slow-moving and is a good place for beginners to start. Ashtanga Yoga is intense and physically demanding so will increase your fitness. Hot Yoga is practiced in a heated room to loosen your muscles and encourage sweating.

## Fish Oil

Humans have been trying to relieve pain since we came to be. Religious practices like making sacrifices and scaring away 'spirits' that were causing the pain were a popular choice thousands of years ago. We now have many much more reliable methods of pain management available.

One that you might not be aware of is simple fish oil. It can be effective at reducing back or neck pain, as one study of 250 people showed. 60% of people reported that their pain had decreased while taking fish oil and 80% said they would continue to take the supplement for this reason.

Fish oil can be a safer alternative to traditional pharmaceutical painkillers like ibuprofen. It has fewer unwanted side effect, as well as providing many other health benefits when taken.

## Heat Therapy

Temperature changes are often used to try and improve different health conditions. Heat therapy is a good option for pain treatment, including lower back and neck pain. A heated blanket or heat wrap provides short term pain relief while being used. Studies have also shown that using a heat wrap while exercising can reduce your pain even more.

*Take care with heat therapy! It is easy to overdo it and suffer from burns or blisters.*

Different styles of heat wraps are available. Some are disposable, others can be reused. There are those designed to wrap around your middle section and stay put without you needing to touch then, leaving your hands free to get on with your life. Other types of heat treatments include hot water bottles, hot towels, hot baths or saunas and infra-red lamps.

## Glucosamine

After vitamins or minerals, Glucosamine is the next most commonly taken supplement. Glucosamine is an amino sugar, this means it is usually made inside your body and is used to build proteins that your body needs.

Taking a Glucosamine supplement may be helpful for reducing knee pain, both in people with and without osteoarthritis. A study showed that after

3 months of treatment, people who took glucosamine daily had less pain and were able to complete their daily activities more easily.

Glucosamine is not found in many food sources. The best way to increase your intake of it is to take a supplement. The glucosamine in these supplements are usually extracted from the shells of shrimps, lobsters or crabs.

## Music Therapy

Making and listening to music has been part of the human way of life for a long, long time. The earliest instrument, which could be described as a type of flute made of bone, is estimated to have been made almost 40,000 years ago. Music is such an important part of our lives, it is not surprising that it may be able to help our health.

Listening to music can reduce your pain. A study showed that people who listened to music while recovering from surgery reported less pain and needed fewer painkillers than people who did not.

*You do not need to be a musician or have musical experience to benefit from music therapy, it does not involve teaching an instrument or learning to sing better! Sometimes singing can cause others pain especially on certain American TV Programmes.*

It was once thought that only 'high-brow, sophisticated' music would be effective at reducing pain, but in the study there was no difference between people who listened to music the scientists picked for them or those who chose their own music.

## UV

Ultra Violet (UV) light is a type of light we cannot see, because the waves are too short to be picked up by our eyes. Sunlight contains UV light but most of it is filtered out by the atmosphere that surrounds the earth, before it can get to you.

UV light may be effective at reducing pain in your body. People with fibromyalgia who were exposed to extra UV light on a tanning bed for six weeks had a happier outlook on life and reduced pain after just two weeks.

All tanning beds contain UV lamps as UV is the type of light that causes your skin to turn brown. You should be able to find a local beauty salon with a tanning bed or can purchase your own lamp. It is suggested that you use them once a week to help with pain. However be careful of long term use, as UV light may be a cause of skin cancer.

## Pine Bark

When French Maritime pine trees were introduced to South Africa 150 years ago, they grew so quickly and took over such a large amount of land in a short space of time that they are now considered a problem.

Pine bark extract, often known by the brand name Pycnogenol, may be a good way to treat period pain in women. Over 100 women who experienced pain ranging from a few cramps to full-out dysmenorrhea participated in a study that showed taking Pycnogenol soothed their pain and reduced their need for other painkillers. On average the number of painful days decreased from 2.1 to 1.3.

*Dysmenorrhea is the medical term for the painful cramps that may occur immediately before or during the menstrual cycle.*

Pycnogenol and other supplements containing pine bark extract are available for you to buy. It's not recommended that you try to eat the tree itself!

## Vitamin D

Being fat-soluble, vitamin D is carried through your body in your blood. It goes through changes in your liver and then your kidneys and comes out as calcitriol (the form of vitamin D that your body uses).

Not getting enough vitamin D was linked to chronic pain in a study of almost 7,000 people. Women who got the most vitamin D both from their food and spending time outdoors were least likely to suffer from a chronic pain disorder. This only applied to women though, pain in men seemed unaffected by vitamin D levels.

Sunlight is the easiest way to get your daily dose of vitamin D. The amount of time you need to spend outdoors depends on your skin colour and age. Lighter skinned people need less time than those with darker skin and more exposure is needed as your grow older. Always avoid staying in the sun too long, as you increase your chance of sunburn and risk skin cancer.

## Antioxidants

Chronic pancreatitis is a serious problem that causes acute pain. It happens when your pancreas stops working as it should and your body can't properly absorb nutrients from food. Antioxidants might be helpful at lowering the pain you feel from chronic pancreatitis.

*The pancreas is a long, flat organ which is tucked in behind the stomach in the upper abdomen. Many people do not know what it does. It makes enzymes that help food digestion and hormones that help regulate the way your body processes sugar.*

A study showed that after 6 months of taking antioxidant supplements regularly, the average number of days where people were in pain due to pancreatitis more than halved. The number of painkillers they needed also dropped by about the same amount. Some people even reported that they were pain free.

Antioxidants can be found in lots of fresh food, including most fruit, vegetables and herbs. Getting your 5+ servings of fruit and vegetables a day is an easy way of making sure you have heaps of antioxidants flowing around your body. Berries, artichokes and kale are particularly loaded with them.

## Baths

Balneotherapy is the official name for the practice of using baths to help treat an illness. It has been a popular treatment in Europe and Japan for centuries, and is beginning to gain recognition worldwide. A nice hot bath is often just what you feel like when you are in pain and the evidence suggests there is a good reason for this.

Studies have found that 'bath therapy' can help relieve pain in people with fibromyalgia. It decreased the number of painful 'pressure points' on their bodies and improved their mood.

Baths can just be hot water baths or they can have minerals, herbs or essential oils added to the water. Balneotherapists are health professionals with experience in bath therapy and they can help you to discover the combination that works best for you.

## Physical Manipulation

Osteotherapy and chiropractic treatment are both complementary therapies that focus on the relationship between your bones, muscles and general health. Their underlying principle is that if your bones and muscles are well positioned and looked after, then your body will be able to function better and heal well.

This may be true in the case of fibromyalgia with studies showing that both types of treatment helped reduce pain. Physical manipulation also helped with other symptoms of fibromyalgia including reducing fatigue, improving the ability to move generally, completing daily activities and lifting mood.

*Not much is known about fibromyalgia and it is one of the most difficult conditions for doctors to treat. It is a disease whose main symptoms are widespread musculoskeletal pain, often with fatigue, sleep, memory and mood problems as well.*

Osteotherapy and chiropractic treatment should only be done by a qualified professional. Your doctor may be able to refer you to a practitioner in your local area.

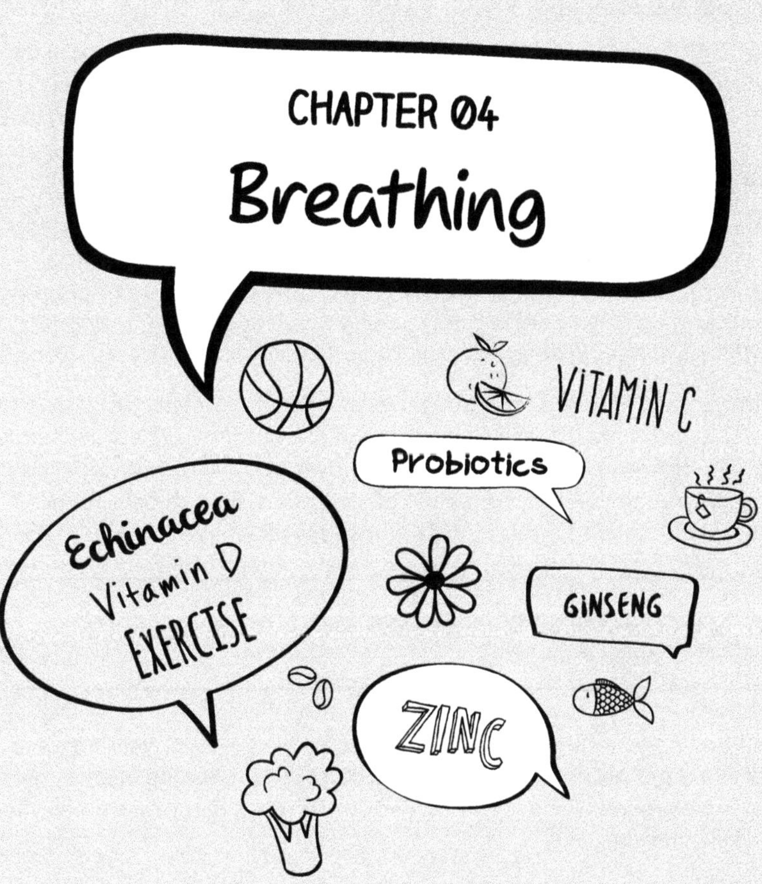
CHAPTER 04
Breathing
VITAMIN C
Probiotics
Echinacea
Vitamin D
EXERCISE
GINSENG
ZINC

It's something you learnt to do almost the second you were born, yet stuffy noses or allergic reactions can make even this simple act seem difficult sometimes. This chapter will cover two issues related to breathing; the common cold and asthma.

Around 1 in 12 people suffer from asthma. Hippocrates was the first person to recognize and name the disease in around 450 B.C. The word asthma comes from the Greek language, and simply means '*difficulty breathing*'. Asthma is caused by your airways narrowing, making it more difficult for air to go in and out.

Usually, this is triggered by an allergic reaction to something you have breathed in, such as smoke, pollen, dust or mould. The number of people who suffer from asthma is increasing each year, as is the number of people dying from asthma. This is not just happening in developing countries, but worldwide including places such as the United States.

A cold affects each of us around three times a year and normally just lasts a few days, but each time it happens you run the risk of triggering a more serious infection. The common cold can be caused by over 400 different culprits and they come with an unpleasant collection of symptoms. Sore throats, runny noses, and tiredness are all the norm for this easily caught sickness.

*Did you know that when you sneeze, contagious germs can be spread up to six feet away from you?*

It's not all bad news though, the number of colds we get each year tends to decrease as we get older, the reason being that with increasing age we have already been exposed to more and more of the viruses that cause colds and have become immune.

## Ginseng

Ginseng is a plant that comes in two varieties, Asian ginseng and American ginseng. In Traditional Chinese medicine American ginseng is said to increase yin (shadows and coolness), while Asian ginseng is thought to increase yang (sunshine and heat). American ginseng has traditionally been used to 'cool' infections and fevers.

The cooling properties of American ginseng can be a great help in boosting your immune system. A study has found that taking ginseng can reduce your likelihood of getting a cold by 30%, and can make any colds you do catch milder. The root is the part typically used in medicines. While it is occasionally eaten, it can also be drunk as a tea or taken as a supplement.

## Echinacea

Echinacea is a type of purple daisy that blooms from early to late summer. Its ability to fight the common cold is widely recognised. It stimulates your body's immune system, making it better able to fight off infections should you come into contact with someone who is contagious. Information taken from many studies about echinacea's ability to combat colds has been looked at in a systematic review.

*A systematic review is when researchers look at all of the studies that have been undertaken for a certain treatment for a condition and draw conclusions. The findings are therefore stronger than those from a single study.*

Taking echinacea can lower your risk of catching a cold by 58% and can shorten the length of your cold by almost one and a half days.

The best way to take echinacea is in a capsule form. These are readily available over the counter at pharmacies or health stores. Echinacea should be avoided by people with various autoimmune diseases, as its ability to impact the immune system may have harmful effects.

*Warning: people with asthma are advised to be careful as in rare cases echinacea can cause severe, life-threatening allergic reactions.*

## Vitamin D

Rickets, is a disease that causes soft bones in children, so soft that they could not support them. This was a risk due to not getting enough vitamin D. This disease is now rare in developed countries, thank goodness! Vitamin D has since been recognised for its uses other than growing strong bones.

High vitamin D levels in your blood lower your chances of getting a cold or other infection in the top part of the respiratory system, caused by viruses and bacteria. A 19,000 person study strongly linked people with low levels of vitamin D with an increased risk of catching this type of cold.

Most of your vitamin D will probably come from sunlight. Some food has vitamin D added to make it as easy as possible to get your required intake. Natural sources of vitamin D include oily fish, cheese and egg yolks.

## Zinc

The first known use of zinc was 2500 years ago, Ancient Greek ornaments were made of a combination of zinc and other metals. It is now known to be an essential mineral for general health, with there being more of it than any other trace element in your body (except iron).

Low levels of zinc can cause your immune system to not be able to properly fight off colds. A study found that when zinc lozenges were sucked regularly, people had shorter colds and the symptoms were not as severe.

The best sources of zinc is from natural unprocessed food. Red meat (lamb and beef), whole grain food, oysters and nuts are all great additions to your diet if you want to increase your zinc levels.

*Warning: Large doses of zinc should be avoided if you are pregnant.*

## Exercise

Walking, running, swimming, cycling, team sports; however you like your exercise, you probably already know how good it is for you. There is a link between exercise and your risk of catching a cold.

In a study, women who exercised for 45 minutes five days a week were three times less likely to get colds than those who only exercised for 45 minutes once a week. The exercise they did was 'moderate intensity.' This includes exercise such as brisk walking, playing tennis, pushing a lawnmower or even other chores around the house where you are standing or crouching.

Exercising while you are sick will not reduce the length of your cold, but it may give you more energy and clear your head for a short amount of time.

*When deciding whether or not to exercise when ill, a good rule of thumb is that if all your symptoms are above your neck, then you're probably good to go.*

## Probiotics

Probiotics are good bacteria that work in your digestive system, breaking down food and releasing the vitamins you need. They also help your immune system to keep going strong and may reduce your risk of getting an infection.

*A lot of people do not know that our gastrointestinal tract is home to about seventy percent of the immune system.*

A study of very ill people who needed help breathing from a ventilator found that those who received probiotic bacteria were less likely to get an infection than those who received standard treatments.

A range of probiotic rich yoghurts are available, but the level of probiotics in these is quite low. For a stronger dose, probiotic supplements are available.

## Vitamin E

Vitamin E was first used as a medicine in 1938 for premature babies who were not growing properly. Over half the babies who received it went on to grow normally. Vitamin E is an antioxidant that comes in eight different forms, with each form found in a different type of food.

In a study of almost 1900 expectant mothers, having lots of vitamin E in your diet while pregnant, makes your child less likely to develop asthma or have breathing difficulties after they are born.

Vitamin E is not naturally made in your body, and you can only get it by eating vitamin E rich food or taking a supplement. Nuts and seeds such as sunflower seeds, almonds, and hazelnuts are easy to snack on and have high levels of vitamin E. Other food sources include green leafy vegetables, kiwifruit, avocados, whole grains, eggs, milk, dairy products and meat. If taking a supplement look for the natural 'd-alpha' vitamin E, the synthetic version is 'dl-alpha'.

## Magnesium

We all have around 25 grams of magnesium in our body at any time, most of it in our bones and skeletal muscle. Magnesium is an essential element in the life and death of the sun and other stars, but it is also essential in keeping another star healthy - you! Magnesium can also be used as a treatment for children suffering from asthma.

A study gave severely asthmatic children magnesium supplements. These children had fewer asthma attacks, needed less asthma medication and had fewer allergic reactions compared to the children who did not have magnesium supplements.

Magnesium is found naturally in green leafy vegetables, meat, starches, grains, nuts and milk. It can also be taken as a supplement and there are many forms. The cheaper magnesium oxide may not be well absorbed if you have stomach issues.

## Vitamin C

Oranges are a common remedy to ward off colds and infections because they are a great source of vitamin C. Vitamin C can help prevent you catching a cold after a hard workout session or being caught out in the rain.

A study showed that taking vitamin C when there is a risk of getting sick, can halve your chance of actually catching a cold. If you do get sick it can also decrease the length of your cold, so long as you had been taking vitamin C before the symptoms appeared.

Exercising can make asthma symptoms worse, but vitamin C could help reduce the effect it has on your breathing. People with asthma who took a vitamin C supplement were less likely to suffer from exercise-induced bronchoconstriction.

*Bronchoconstriction is a contraction, or tightening of the airways (breathing tubes) which causes the shortness of breath and wheezing which are the hallmarks of asthma.*

## Caffeine

This is one remedy you will almost certainly have heard of. Cocoa, or hot chocolate, was the first caffeinated drink to make its way into western culture as early as the 1500s. Tea and coffee weren't drunk by Europeans until almost a century later.

Caffeine can reduce symptoms of asthma: it makes your body release adrenaline, the get-up-and-go hormone that widens your airways. A study showed that people who were given caffeine had less difficulty breathing, an improvement much the same as those people who were given the common asthma drug, theophylline.

Caffeine is easy to come across, being found in coffee, tea, caffeinated soft drinks and chocolate. In the unlikely event that you are not a fan of any of these, or want to increase your dose, tablet and powder forms are available.

*Warning too much caffeine can be very dangerous (even fatal) in extremely high doses and can cause jitteriness, sleeplessness, stomach irritation, nausea and vomiting.*

## Antioxidants

Oxidation, in your body, is when a substance goes around stealing small particles of atoms known as electrons from other parts of your body. This can damage the molecules, cells and tissues that they get stolen from and can cause that area to become swollen and sore.

Antioxidants help to keep this oxidation in control. They reduce swelling inside your body, which can help lessen the symptoms and conditions of asthma. A study found that children who ate food with more antioxidants were less likely to have difficulty breathing.

Citrus fruit has lots of antioxidants in them. In a study people who ate more than 45 grams of citrus fruit per day had a reduced risk of getting asthma. To put this in perspective, an orange is around 130 grams and half a cup of chopped pineapple is around 120 grams. Nuts are also healthy snacks that contain plenty of antioxidants.

## Omega-3

Omega-3 fatty acid is one type of fat that you don't want to cut out of your diet. It works as an anti-inflammatory and can help you fight illnesses caused by inflammation or swelling. Omega-3 fatty acids can be used to prevent or treat asthma.

Several studies have shown that high levels of omega-3 improve your ability to breathe efficiently. A different study has shown that children who receive omega-3 supplements have less asthma symptoms than children who do not.

The best source of omega-3 fatty acids are oily fish. The oilier the fish, the more fatty acids it has. Salmon, herring and anchovies are all great choices to increase your omega-3 levels. Walnuts and flaxseed also contain high levels.

## Pine Tree Bark - Pycnogenol

Pycnogenol is a bark extract that has anti-inflammatory properties and helps boost your immune system. It is taken from French Maritime Pine trees, which can grow up to 100 feet tall and have red-brown bark. It can be taken to potentially lessen your asthma symptoms.

Several studies have found that people who took a Pycnogenol supplement were able to breathe more easily and had less asthma symptoms than people who did not.

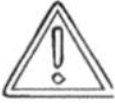

*Warning: As Pycnogenol increases the activity of your immune system, it may worsen the symptoms of multiple sclerosis, coeliac disease and other autoimmune diseases.*

Pycnogenol can only be taken as an oral supplement. Grape seed extract also contains a similar blend of antioxidants.

## Green Tea

Caffeinated drinks are often not associated with being able to help you sleep, but in this case there may be an exception. Green tea might protect your brain if you suffer from a breathing disorder while you sleep.

Sleep apnea and other related conditions cause you to miss breaths during your sleep and can deprive your brain of oxygen. You might also frequently wake yourself up by stopping breathing in your sleep and this can be exhausting. Studies have shown that taking a green tea extract can reduce the damage to your brain and help you get a better night's sleep.

If you choose to go for a supplement, have a look at the caffeine content on the label otherwise it might stop you being able to sleep at all! A hot cup of green tea before bed might be a good way to get the benefits.

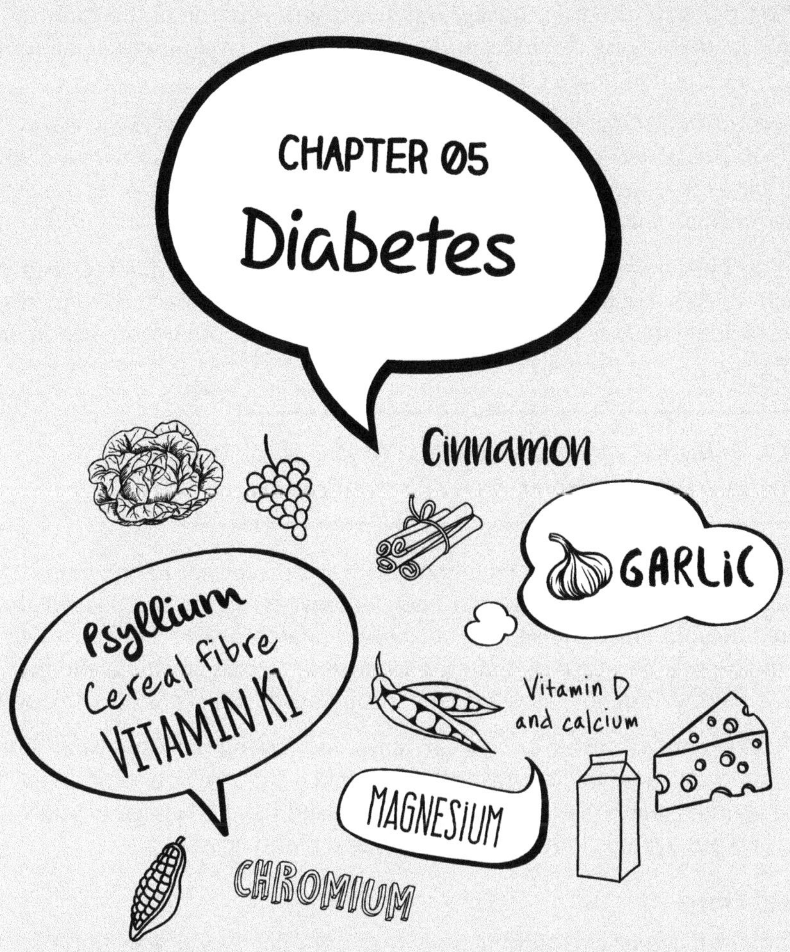
CHAPTER 05
Diabetes
Cinnamon
GARLIC
Psyllium
Cereal fibre
VITAMIN K1
Vitamin D
and calcium
MAGNESIUM
CHROMIUM

Over 400 million people worldwide have diabetes. Its full name, diabetes mellitus, comes from the Greek language and in English translates to '*passing a lot of urine that tastes like honey.*' This sweetness was one of the earliest symptoms identifying diabetics in the past, with ancient Romans and ancient Indians seeing if ants were attracted to the liquid.

Doctors in the 1700s went as far as to taste a patient's urine! Even now health professionals still test urine for excess sugar to see if someone might have diabetes, but these days they use test strips that have special chemicals on them which change colour.

Diabetes has two main types. 10% of diabetics have type 1 diabetes and the remaining 90% have type 2. In both types, diabetes is characterised by high levels of sugar in your blood. Type 1 occurs when your body stops producing insulin.

*Insulin is the hormone responsible for turning sugar in your blood into a different form of 'stored' energy.*

Type 1 normally develops in childhood, with symptoms appearing quite quickly. With type 2 diabetes, your body still makes insulin, but it is mostly ignored by your body and so cannot change sugar into stored energy as well as it did before. This type of diabetes occurs mostly only in adults and the symptoms develop more slowly as the insulin produced is gradually ignored.

Not having enough stored energy can leave you feeling tired and weak. But the main problem with diabetes is that too much sugar in your blood can cause serious health risks, including an increased risk of damage to your eyes, nervous system, kidneys, heart, skin and blood vessels.

## Cereal Fibre

Sometimes it seems like nothing more than your doctor's slogan, but a healthy balanced diet really can prevent a multitude of illnesses. You can lower your risk of getting type 2 diabetes by making sure you eat plenty of fibre, found in fruit, vegetables and whole grain food.

A study showed that people who ate bread fortified with added fibre, were better able to control the levels of sugar in their blood than people who ate simple white bread.

*There are two types of fibre that your body needs: soluble and insoluble. Both come from plants and are forms of carbohydrates. Soluble fibre absorbs water, turning into a mush (eg. oatmeal) while insoluble fibre doesn't (eg. celery).*

You don't necessarily need any supplements to make sure you get enough fibre, it can easily be done by cutting back on highly processed food such as desserts, chips and ready-made snacks. Instead, try vegetables in a range of different colours and pick up the brown/whole wheat variety of flour, rice and pasta at the supermarket. Kidney beans and lentils are also a great source of fibre that can easily be added to a meal.

## Omega-3

No one remembers the taste of cod liver oil fondly, but there are a range of liquids and capsules that can be taken to increase your omega-3 levels, without the horrible aftertaste. Omega-3 is well known for its ability to lower the risk of heart disease. People with type 1 and type 2 diabetes both have an increased risk of heart disease and so it can be taken to lower this risk.

It can also be taken by children who have a higher chance of developing type 1 diabetes when they are very young. A five year study followed children who were considered likely to get type 1 diabetes. Those children who took omega-3 supplements had a lower chance of being diagnosed with type 1 diabetes.

## Garlic

Garlic has been used to treat illnesses for centuries, with its use being recorded in ancient Egyptian, Greek, Roman, Chinese and Indian texts. Recent studies have shown that raw garlic can be effective at preventing heart disease and lowering blood sugar levels.

If you like the taste (and can deal with the resulting bad breath!) garlic can be added to many homemade dishes. If you aren't such a fan supplements, including odourless ones, are available.

*Warning: Pregnant or breastfeeding women may want to avoid garlic, as it can cause heartburn or even affect the taste of their milk. Garlic can thin the blood (reduce the ability of blood to clot), so beware of this if you are about to have surgery or if you take any medicines that can thin the blood such as warfarin.*

## Magnesium

Magnesium is not just a vague memory from high-school science, but an important mineral for your body to work properly. Not having enough magnesium in your diet can stop your body being able to control your blood sugar levels. This happens as less insulin is made and your body ignores more of the insulin in your blood.

A study followed over 4,000 women and the food they ate for eight years. Women who ate less magnesium-rich food were more likely to get type 2 diabetes than those who had more magnesium in their diet.

Increasing your magnesium levels is easy, as magnesium is found in many commonly eaten types of food.

*Chocolate lovers will be pleased to know that magnesium is also found in cocoa!*

Green leafy vegetables, meat, seafood, nuts, whole grain food and milk all have high levels of magnesium. For a quick simple snack, apples, apricots and bananas all contain plenty of magnesium.

## Vitamin D

Slip, slop, slap and wrap - a great slogan for preventing skin cancer, but it may also be preventing you from getting enough vitamin D. Many studies have shown that most people do not have enough vitamin D.

Getting plenty of vitamin D lowers your risk of developing type 2 diabetes by over 300%. Children and teenagers with type 1 diabetes also need to be aware of their vitamin D levels, as studies have shown that over three quarters of them do not have enough.

Low levels of vitamin D can stop your body absorbing enough calcium, causing problems with bones in later life and an increased risk of them breaking.

Spending more time outdoors isn't the only way to increase your vitamin D. Food like oily fish and cheese naturally contain high levels of vitamin D. You can also buy food such as cereal or dairy products with it added and a variety of vitamin D supplements are available and most multivitamins contain vitamin D3.

## Vitamin K1

Vitamin K1 is essential in helping blood clot, stopping you bleeding when you get cut, (doctors call it the clotting vitamin). It is not typically taken as a supplement, but new-born babies often get a one-off injection as they do not have enough of it after birth.

For men aged 60 or over, vitamin K1 lowers the risk of developing diabetes. A study showed that older men with high levels of vitamin K1 were better able to control their blood sugar levels as vitamin K increases the body's response to insulin. It is unclear why vitamin K1 only did this in older men.

*People who may be low in Vitamin Kl include people with a poor or restricted diet, people with conditions that interfere with nutrient absorption such as Crohn's disease and people with liver diseases.*

All of the green leafy vegetables such as spinach, cabbage and (everyone's favourite) brussel sprouts are great sources of vitamin K1.

## Ginseng

This is a slow-growing plant with fleshy roots that has long been used in traditional Chinese medicine. Ginseng prefers cooler climates and grows in North America and Eastern Asia. Studies show that ginseng extracts lower blood sugar levels and that it can be used to lower blood sugar after a meal or long-term if taken daily.

While ginseng can be added to dishes such as soups, the best way to ensure you get enough to receive the benefits is to take it as a supplement. While American or 'true' Ginseng is native to Northern America it is now also widely cultivated in China.

## Pine Bark Extract - Pycnogenol

Pycnogenol, also called pine bark extract, is a supplement that contains an extract from the bark of 20 to 25 year old French Maritime Pine trees. It has many reported uses in medicine, potentially helping with problems ranging from asthma and allergy relief to heart disease. For diabetes patients, it can help protect you from many problems associated with diabetes and can be used to help lower blood sugar levels.

Advanced diabetes symptoms can include loss of eyesight, nerve/blood vessel damage and skin ulcers. Studies have shown that Pycnogenol can be used to treat all of these complications. It can be taken as a pill, or as a cream that is rubbed onto affected areas. Both have been found to be effective with using a combination of both having the best results.

Pycnogenol has low toxicity and mild side effects, but has the potential to interact with other drugs, so it is important to discuss its use (and any supplements you use) with your health professional.

## Alpha-Lipoic Acid

You may know that the mitochondria is known as the powerhouse of the cell, but did you know that Alpha-Lipoic Acid (ALA) is one of the powerhouse chemicals inside the mitochondria itself? ALA along with other chemicals makes the energy-producing reactions within the cells happen.

Many studies have shown that ALA can help lower blood sugar, by making your body more responsive to insulin. It has also been shown to help with nerve damage that can occur in advanced diabetes.

You can get your ALA through food such as liver and yeast, or it can be taken as a supplement.

## Psyllium

The seeds and husks of the psyllium plant are covered with a gummy substance that thickens when it enters your intestines. This helps to control blood sugar levels, as the thickening slows the digestion and the speed at which the sugar from your food is absorbed into your blood.

In studies, people taking psyllium had lower blood sugar levels after meals than people who were not taking it. It also reduces the amount of fat you absorb from your food, potentially reducing your risk of heart disease.

Psyllium is sometimes found in breads, cereal and muesli bars.

*Common brand names for psyllium are Metamucil, Konsyl and Reguloid.*

It can also be taken as a variety of different forms of supplement, including just eating the seeds or in capsules and tablets.

## Chromium

Chromium is an essential mineral your body needs to help regulate blood sugar. It works together with insulin to turn sugar into energy in your body. Low levels of chromium can prevent insulin from working properly, which causes increased levels of sugar in your blood.

Studies suggest that taking chromium can decrease blood sugar levels in people with type 1, type 2 or pregnancy related diabetes. It has also proven to be helpful at lowering cholesterol in your blood.

It is found in small amounts in food like broccoli, green beans, grape juice, orange juice and mashed potatoes. Supplements can also be taken and it is usually present in any good multivitamin.

## Cinnamon

This spice has many uses, having been used for centuries in flavourings, ancient medicines and for its sweet spicy smell. It is native to Sri Lanka and Southern India and the bark is thought to prevent colds, infections and upset stomachs.

A study has shown that it can be taken to reduce blood sugar levels in people with type 2 diabetes, as well as lower cholesterol levels.

You may already enjoy a sprinkling of cinnamon on your coffee every now and again, but this is probably not enough to get any health benefits. You would have to eat approximately 2 teaspoons of cinnamon a day to get the full dose used in the study. So unless you really have a taste for this spice, supplemental cinnamon is probably your only option.

## Fenugreek

Fenugreek was first used by the ancient Egyptians in the embalming of their dead and fenugreek seeds have even been found inside the tomb of the young pharaoh, King Tutankhamun. Currently it is used to treat a variety of illnesses and can be used to help control blood sugar levels in people with type 2 diabetes.

Studies have shown that it can increase how well insulin works in your body, as well as lowering blood sugar levels after just 10 days.

Fenugreek is found in some mixed spice blends and can be used as a flavouring ingredient in some dishes. You can also take it as a supplement, in the form of capsules, powder or even tea.

## Guar Gum

The guar plant is native to India and its gum is used in food manufacturing as a thickener and binding agent. When it enters your intestines it expands and absorbs water and has been used to treat both constipation and diarrhoea in the past.

Studies have shown that guar gum can also lower your blood sugar levels and your cholesterol levels. In one study, people who ate a breakfast containing guar gum had lower blood sugar levels after their meal, than people who did not.

*Some people are allergic to guar gum and can have reactions to it such as flushing, itchiness and diarrhoea.*

Guar gum can be taken as a powder, tablet or in granule form. As guar gum absorbs water it is important to stay well hydrated when taking it. There is also a risk that it could absorb other medications you are taking, so be sure to check with your healthcare provider before you begin taking this supplement.

## Fibre and Magnesium

Both of these substances have already been given a mention in this chapter, but taken together they have a powerful ability to reduce the risk of developing type 2 diabetes. This was demonstrated in a study of over 25,000 people who were at risk of developing diabetes. When added up, the study collected data which was equivalent to a total of 200,000 years and the conclusion was that an increased amount of fibre and magnesium in the diet lowered the chance of getting type 2 diabetes.

Helpfully, food rich in fibre also tend to contain plenty of magnesium. Whole grains, seeds, nuts and legumes like kidney beans and lentils are all excellent sources of both fibre and magnesium.

## Vitamin D and Calcium

Calcium helps build strong, robust bones, with 99% of the calcium in your body being found in your bones and teeth. A combination of vitamin D and calcium supplements may lower the risk of getting type 2 diabetes in people who are at high risk of developing the disease.

Studies have shown an association between low levels of vitamin D, low dairy intake and increased chance of having type 2 diabetes.

Calcium can be found in all dairy products, such as milk, yoghurt, and cheese. Leafy greens are also a good source of calcium, with kale and broccoli containing high levels of it. Sometimes calcium is added to fruit juice, tofu and cereal. And, you guessed it, supplements are also available and they can contain just calcium, or both calcium and vitamin D.

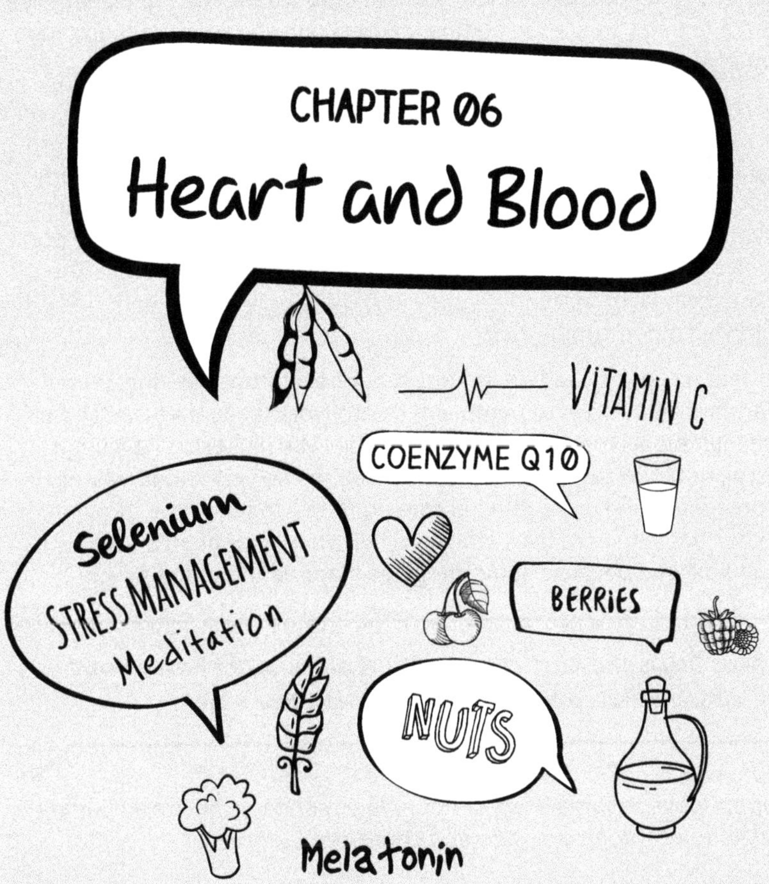
CHAPTER 06
Heart and Blood
VITAMIN C
COENZYME Q10
Selenium
STRESS MANAGEMENT
Meditation
BERRIES
NUTS
Melatonin

The heart is an organ that has the same purpose in almost all animals, to pump blood around the body. Jelly fish, sea sponges and starfish are the only animals without one. The largest heart in the animal kingdom weighs in at almost 700 kilograms and belongs to the blue whale. Most of us have red blood but a few sea species including lobsters and shrimp have blood that is bright blue! This is because they have copper in their blood.

Your heart is a pretty important part of you. It started beating when you were just four weeks old in your mother's womb and by the time you were born it was pumping the equivalent of one cup of blood throughout your body. Now, your heart is probably pumping an average of around five litres of blood every minute. Your blood must be pumped through around 100,000 kilometres of blood vessels to reach almost every part of your body. The cornea, the clear layer in front of your eyes, is the only part of your body that doesn't have a blood supply to it.

It's clear that it is pretty bad news when your heart stops working. When your heart finds it difficult to pump and has to work really hard each beat, you have high blood pressure. Sometimes this is because you have high cholesterol, or blood fat levels. If fat builds up inside your blood vessels it can become more and more difficult for your heart to pump the blood and oxygen your body needs. Heart attacks occur when your heart suddenly can't get enough oxygen because something has stopped the blood flow.

*Christmas Day is the most common day that you might have a heart attack, closely followed by Boxing Day and New Year's Eve.*

This chapter looks at some ways to improve your heart's health, including therapies to lower blood pressure and cholesterol levels.

## Calcium and Vitamin D

Coming from the Latin word '*calx*' meaning lime, calcium was used by the Romans as lime (what we now know as calcium chloride) in their buildings in the first century. Calcium and vitamin D are two supplements that work together. Both are necessary for the other to work and as a team, they have some excellent benefits. They can lower your cholesterol levels and make you less likely to suffer from heart disease.

A study of obese women showed that taking them improved total, LDL and HDL cholesterol levels.

*LDL (low-density lipoprotein cholesterol) is also called 'bad' cholesterol and high levels are bad for us. HDL (high-density lipoprotein cholesterol), is also called 'good' cholesterol and high levels are good for us.*

When you have congestive heart failure, your heart doesn't pump properly and your blood pools in places it shouldn't. This makes your limbs swell up uncomfortably. Taking vitamin D and calcium can help, as it might lower the amount of chemicals in your blood responsible for the swelling.

## Vitamin C

Most animals can make their own vitamin C, but not us humans. Along with monkeys, bats and guinea pigs, we lost this ability somewhere back in our evolutionary history. Vitamin C has so many health benefits that this is rather a shame.

Reducing bad cholesterol in the blood is one important way that vitamin C helps your body. An analysis of 13 studies showed that the level of harmful blood cholesterol goes down when the level of vitamin C goes up.

You may believe that citrus fruit is the best source of vitamin C and you wouldn't be the only one. However it is actually a vegetable, the capsicum (bell pepper) that is the best source as it contains one and a half times the amount of vitamin C as the same sized portion of citrus fruit does.

## Berries

Strawberries are the only fruit that has its seeds on the outside. There are over 200 tiny seeds on each strawberry. As well as being delicious, berries contain polyphenols. These are a part of the plant's defence mechanism and act as an antioxidant when inside your body.

Eating lots of berries can help lower your cholesterol, your blood pressure and can help to stop unwanted blood clots. A two month study showed that regular consumption of lots of different types of berries might help lower your risk of heart disease.

While fresh summer berries have to be the most appealing, you don't have to stop eating berries once winter begins. Frozen berries can be just as tasty and still contain all the antioxidants you need. Try keeping a variety of berries in your freezer to throw into a breakfast smoothie or eat them as a frozen dessert.

## Flavonoids

Flavonoids make up the largest nutrient family currently known and contain over 6,000 different types. They are split into different categories depending on their particular effect on your body. Different types of flavonoids are found in fruit, vegetables and some drinks.

An analysis of over 130 studies showed that they may lower blood pressure and levels of bad cholesterol.

Flavonoids found in chocolate and soy protein might well be good at reducing your risk of heart disease. To get the type of flavonoids used in many of the research studies, eating dark chocolate is one way to go. The higher the percentage of cocoa, the more flavonoids it contains.

## Hawthorn

A tree in France has a small plaque which reads '*This hawthorn is probably the oldest tree in France*'. It claims to date back to the third century. It is impossible to know if this is true, but even so it is an impressive claim. Age isn't the only impressive thing about the hawthorn tree. Taking a hawthorn supplement could help those at risk from chronic heart failure.

At least 14 studies have shown that it can help with physical symptoms of heart problems such as fatigue and shortness of breath. More technical measures of the heart show that it's good for your heart's functioning overall.

Hawthorn extract is a prescription medicine in some countries, which shows how powerful it can be in your body. Make sure you check about drug interactions and other effects with your doctor before you start taking it.

*The main side effects of hawthorn are nausea, stomach upset, dizziness, drowsiness, sweating, trouble sleeping, and headaches.*

## Selenium

Once popular for its use in electronics, selenium has now been replaced by silicon in most circuit systems. It's commonly used in baby formula and also in dandruff shampoo. In your body, it works as an antioxidant and you might benefit if you suffer from heart disease.

Over 400 people participated in a study that showed the more you took, the greater the antioxidant effects were in people with coronary artery disease.

*Low selenium levels in soil mean that around one third of males and over half of females do not get enough selenium.*

A couple of brazil nuts a day is all you need to get the selenium you need. Other food sources high in selenium include eggs, meat and seafood.

## Niacin and Exercise

Not getting enough niacin (vitamin B3) can cause nausea, anaemia, headaches and tiredness. Niacin, when combined with exercise, can be a great supplement for lowering blood cholesterol and increasing how fast sugar is taken out of your blood and stored. It is seen as one of the most effective treatments for lowering your blood cholesterol and can decrease it by 20-50%.

A study showed that taking a niacin supplement and exercising before a meal can decrease your risk of heart disease.

You are probably well on your way to getting enough niacin if you eat offal (liver and kidney both contain high levels of it). Fish, poultry, mushrooms and sweetcorn are also good sources of niacin. Supplements are also available to take and many doctors in the USA prescribe niacin.

## Meditation

The Transcendental Meditation technique began in the 1950s when Maharishi Mahesh Yogi first introduced it in India and then internationally by a series of world tours. It is a type of mantra meditation that is practised for 15-20 minutes a day. It is a relaxation exercise and might be helpful for people with heart disease.

A study showed that it reduced stress, blood pressure and insomnia while increasing energy levels and memory.

Transcendental Meditation is taught by a certified teacher who will follow a set seven-step course of instruction. It is certainly possible (although studies are limited) that other types of relaxation techniques like yoga and other styles of meditation would be effective as well.

## Compression Stockings

The height of travel fashion, compression stockings do more than just keeping your toes warm on long flights. Deep vein thrombosis (DVT) is a blood clot that can occur in your legs due to bad circulation. Wearing compression stockings can make you 10 times less likely to develop a DVT on long flights. It squeezes the blood out of your calves and back up your legs so that it doesn't pool. DVT's don't always hurt but can be dangerous and even deadly if the clot moves to your lungs or brain.

Long journeys can be hard on your body. Changes in altitude along with sitting down for an extended period of time can be especially tricky if your heart is struggling to pump blood around your body properly under normal circumstances. Other than wearing compression stockings, it's good to keep your blood flowing by taking short walks, bending and straightening your legs and drinking plenty of water.

## Pine Bark

Pine bark extract, commonly known as Pycnogenol, is an antioxidant that is 50 times more potent than vitamin E and 20 times more potent than vitamin C. It might be useful to take a pine bark supplement if you often get leg cramps or muscle pain. Cramps are caused by your muscles not getting enough oxygen.

A study of over 100 people showed that taking pine bark could reduce the pain experienced from cramps.

Pycnogenol is one brand of pine bark extract supplement that you can take and was the one studied in this trial. Side effects can include dizziness and headaches, so keep an eye out for these.

## Melatonin

Your body has an internal clock that keeps track of the passing of time. It reminds us of all sorts of things, from getting hungry at mealtimes, to getting sleepy in the evening. The way this happens is complicated, but we do know that the hormone melatonin is responsible for making us feel tired. Taking melatonin can help lower night time blood pressure by helping the body keep track of what it should be doing and at what time.

Melatonin can be taken as a supplement. Taking it this way allows you to get your dose at the right time and stop you feeling sleepy at inappropriate times. Some food also contains melatonin, including tart cherries, bananas and grapes.

## Vitamin C and Garlic

Garlic is a close relative of the onion, shallot and leek. It has been used by humans for over 7,000 years as both a flavour and a medicine. Increasing your intake of garlic and vitamin C may help lower your blood pressure in as little as 10 days.

A study found that people who had slightly too high blood pressure, saw it decrease to a normal range in just over a week after taking a combination of vitamin c and garlic.

Garlic can be added to many food dishes and is normally fried to help release the flavours, before being added to the rest of the ingredients. Vitamin C is of course found in many varieties of fruit and vegetables, especially capsicums, citrus fruit and green leafy vegetables.

## Green Tea

It is such a common drink in Japan that green tea is simply referred to as 'tea'. It was brought to Japan in the 12th century by a Buddhist priest and since then has become very popular. It is drunk at breakfast, when guests come over and is served for free when you arrive at most restaurants.

A study showed that taking a green tea extract for two months improved both the blood pressure and mood of participants.

Green tea can be drunk as a tea of course, but the amount needed to receive the blood pressure benefits, may be as high as 10 cups a day. You can buy supplements of concentrated green tea, allowing you to get the nutrients quickly and easily.

## Stress Management

You've probably been told that stress isn't good for your health. Your 'flight or fight' response can be helpful to keep out of danger, but if it stays switched on for too long it can be rough on your body. Lowering your stress levels can reduce your blood pressure and might mean you can stop taking any medications you are on to control it.

A study of over 120 people with high blood pressure showed that many of the participants had a decrease in blood pressure after just two months of doing a relaxation training program.

Exercises or techniques to lower your stress levels include yoga, meditation or Tai Chi. The goal is to practice relaxation and make your response to stressful situations more calm and controlled.

## Fish Oil

Back in the 1970s scientists wondered why Eskimos had such a low rate of heart disease despite eating a diet that was so high in fat. It turned out that almost all of the fat they ate was from oily fish.

Since then many, many studies have been done that confirm increasing your oily fish (or omega-3 intake) can lower your risk of bad heart health. It reduces the chance of admission to hospital and death due to heart failure. It does this by decreasing blood pressure, improving heart function and reducing arrhythmias.

*Arrhythmias are abnormal heart rhythms, the most common ones include atrial fibrillation and atrial flutter. In adults more than 100 heart beats per minute is too fast and below 50 beats per minute is too slow.*

Fish oil can stop you from getting heart disease in the first place and can be taken with typical cholesterol lowering drugs like statins to improve their efficiency.

Omega-3 can be taken as a supplement. It is also found in oily fish such as salmon or trout. It is recommended that you eat two to four servings of fish a week to benefit your heart.

## Magnesium

Used in over 300 processes that happen in your body every day, magnesium really is an all-rounder mineral. Making energy, building teeth and keeping your heart pumping are just a few of its important uses. Increasing your magnesium levels makes your heart healthier. A higher intake has been linked to reduced blood pressure, a lower likelihood of getting a stroke, a decreased number of blood clots and better overall heart function.

Studies have also shown that people who have heart disease were able to exercise for longer when they took magnesium.

Dark leafy greens, nuts, seeds and whole grains are all highly recommended if you want more magnesium. It's also plentiful in avocados and bananas, so putting them on whole wheat toast would make an excellent high-magnesium breakfast. Magnesium supplements are also available and your recommended daily intake depends on your weight and changes as you age.

## Alcohol

Humans have been drinking alcohol since fruit juice was left to ferment many centuries ago. It is now a common cultural and social event, more so in some places than others. The French are stereotypically known for drinking large amounts of wine and perhaps this is what leads them to having low rates of heart disease compared to other countries (although studies imply the healthy fats in their diet may be responsible).

Many studies have linked drinking a moderate amount of alcohol (particularly red wine), to a decreased risk of having a heart attack or dying from heart disease.

Most of the studies say that it was *moderate* consumption of alcohol which was linked to the lowest risk of heart disease, but moderate is a subjective term. Some studies recommended a drink every day, whereas others suggested that the optimal amount was a drink on a few nights a week. Remember the other risks you run when drinking alcohol and be careful with your consumption.

## Olive Oil

The olive tree is native to the Mediterranean basin. The first evidence that humans were turning olives into olive oil comes from Israel around 6,000 BC. It was an important part of many cultures, used for religious rituals, medicine, cooking and has even been found in some of the pharaohs tombs in Egypt. It might seem to be a bit of a paradox, but eating olive oil daily can improve the health of your heart and blood. Olive oil is fat, but it is a healthy type of fat which lowers bad cholesterol levels.

Virgin olive oil is one of the best kinds to be consuming. It is made by extraction from the olives and has no chemicals added to it. Olive oil can be a tasty salad dressing on its own or make a great addition to one.

## Nuts

Classed as a fruit with one large seed and a tough layer of flesh, nuts are often seen as high in fat and therefore to be avoided. However this seems to be false information. Many studies have shown that nuts can be effective at lowering your risk of heart disease and reducing your cholesterol levels. Studies show that the more nuts you eat each day, the lower the cholesterol in your blood stream.

Almonds, walnuts, pecans, and peanuts can all be recommended based on the many studies, but all nuts will contain at least some of the nutrients helpful for your heart. Snacking on nuts is satisfying and filling, due in part to the protein content and can make you less likely to snack on other less healthy options.

## Calcium

Plaster of Paris contains a compound of calcium and is used in fast-setting plaster casts when you break a bone. This has been done since the 10th century, when the compound was discovered to be better than the common method of using wooden splints. Calcium has since been discovered to be important for your health in many other ways.

Regular intake of calcium can reduce your risk of having a stroke and studies show that eating plenty of calcium can reduce your blood pressure, especially if you don't normally get enough in your diet.

Eating lots of dairy is one excellent way to increase your calcium intake. Other sources include leafy green vegetables and legumes like beans and chickpeas and of course supplements.

## Coenzyme Q10

95% of the energy your body uses is made in the mitochondria (a part of the cell). Coenzyme Q10 is an important part of this and many other processes in the cells that make up our bodies. It can be taken as a supplement to reduce the muscle pain that is often a side effect of taking statins.

*Statins are a type of medicine often prescribed by doctors in order to help lower cholesterol levels in the blood helping to prevent heart attacks and stroke.*

Studies show that taking coenzyme Q10 can cause people to continue taking statins when they otherwise would have stopped due to the muscle pain it caused them.

It can also help to lower your blood pressure. Studies of people with high blood pressure show that increasing their coenzyme Q10 levels can reduce their blood pressure substantially and in some cases allow them to stop taking their prescribed drugs.

## Psyllium

Fibre is the part of a plant-based food that your body cannot digest. Psyllium is a soluble fibre, which means it turns into a gel when going through your intestines. This slows your digestion down and helps you absorb the nutrients from your food. Increasing your psyllium levels can help to lower your cholesterol.

Many studies have shown that taking psyllium as part of a healthy diet lowers cholesterol more than the healthy diet would by itself.

Psyllium can be found in many high fibre cereals and breads, so increasing your intake may be as simple as swapping to a high fibre brand. You can also buy psyllium flour which you can add to homemade bread or baked treats. Supplements are also available for you to take, but make sure you increase your water intake when taking them.

## Oats

Oats were among the first plants that early humans cultivated. They survive better in colder climates than other crops, which is why countries such as Russia and Canada are the world's largest oat producers. Like psyllium, they contain a type of soluble fibre and so regular consumption of oats may help to lower your cholesterol levels.

Studies show that increasing your intake of oats can lower both your total cholesterol level and the level of bad cholesterol in your body.

Oats can be rolled, crushed or ground into flour. Rolled oats and oat flour are typically used in baking. Breakfast seems to be a good way to get your oats, with crushed oats being the main ingredient in porridge. Many types of muesli also contain oats and so do some granola bars.

## Plant Stanols and Sterols

Phytosterols is the name given to the 200 or so different types of plant chemicals that are molecules chemically related to cholesterol. They are found in the cell membranes of plants, where they play important roles, just like cholesterol does in humans.

Back in the 1950s scientists realised that plant extracts containing these molecules could lower cholesterol levels. They got a bit left behind as many new drugs and supplements began to be discovered but many studies have now proved them to be a useful remedy if you have high cholesterol. One study, conducted by the Mayo Clinic, showed that taking a phytosterol supplement can reduce your level of bad cholesterol by 10%.

*There are two main forms of cholesterol, LDL (low density lipoprotein) and HDL (high density lipoprotein). LDL cholesterol is often referred to as 'bad cholesterol' because too much is unhealthy.*

Phytosterols are found in most plant based food, particularly grains like corn, soy and wheat. Occasionally they are added to food as a health boost, so check the nutrition information on the packaging. You can also get supplements of a variety of phytosterols from your pharmacy.

## Soy

It was first farmed in China and Eastern Asia as long ago as 1,100 BC. Soy is consumed more in Asian countries than the western world, with the average Japanese person eating around 10g of soy a day.

Adding more soy to your diet might reduce your chances of heart disease. Studies show that soy can lower your blood pressure and cause a drop in your cholesterol levels.

Soy comes in many forms. Soy protein is a complete protein that can replace meat in some meals. You could swap out cow's milk for soy milk on your breakfast cereal. Soy nuts are baked soybeans that can be eaten, as a filling, tasty and yet healthy snack. Soy isoflavones, the active ingredient in soy, are also available in a supplement form.

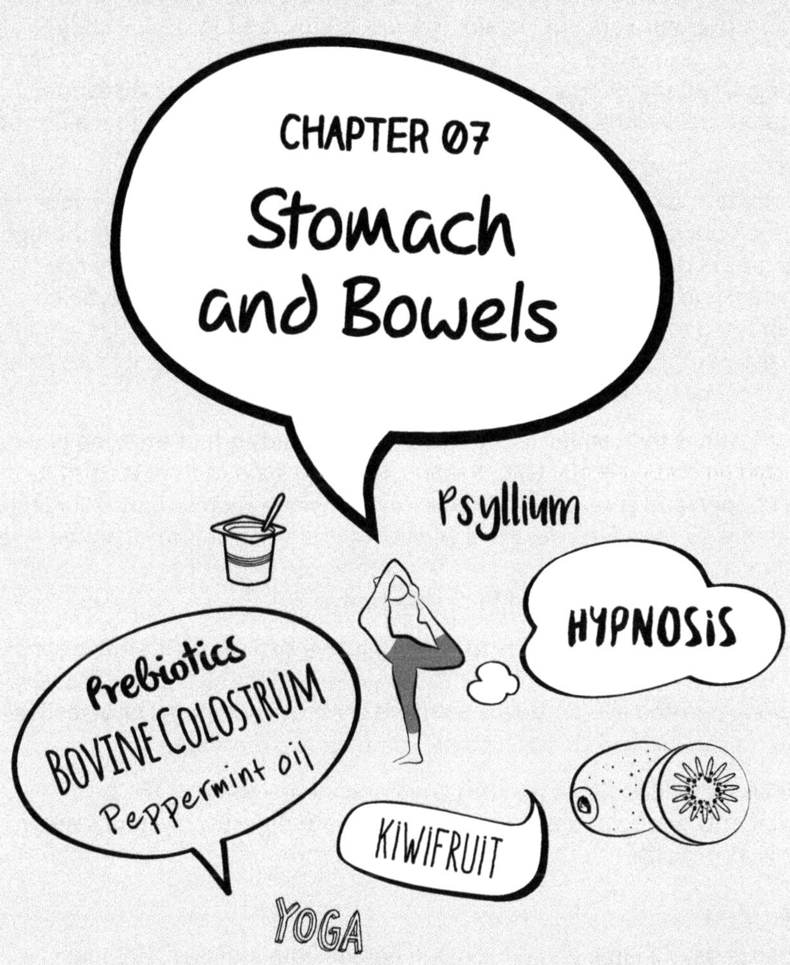
CHAPTER 07
Stomach and Bowels
Psyllium
HYPNOSIS
Prebiotics
BOVINE COLOSTRUM
Peppermint oil
KIWIFRUIT
YOGA

Your digestive system starts with your mouth and ends after several metres of tubing including the stomach and intestines. Every day you eat several meals and maybe some snacks as well (around 1.5-2kg of food), but only around 120grams come out again. The rest is absorbed into your body to be used to make energy or other important things your body needs to keep working. Of all the energy your body uses, 15% is used in the digestion process alone. In other words, you use some of the energy just to make more energy.

Your stomach is the first line of defence against diseases that enter your body via your digestive tract. Acid in your stomach (that could melt through steel) breaks down the food and kills off any nasty germs. Did you know that when you blush, the lining of your stomach also blushes? Maybe it's embarrassed to be heard rumbling so loudly. A rumbling stomach is actually a normal part of the digestive process, it's just that you can hear it more clearly when it echoes around your empty stomach.

Your intestines then squeeze the nutrients and fluids out of the food eaten. Your small intestine really isn't that small at all (it's around 7m long). If it was cut open and spread out it would cover a whole tennis court! Your large intestine is so called because it is wider, but it is much shorter than the small intestine at around 1.5m long. This is where waste matter goes for one last squeeze before being ejected from your body.

There are lots of complex parts to your digestive system, so it's not surprising that there are a variety of things that can go wrong. It's not normally a very nice body part to have problems with and common symptoms of digestive problems can include stomach pains, vomiting and diarrhoea.

You'll be pleased to know that this chapter contains some of the best supplements and remedies to help you and your digestive system stay as healthy as possible.

## Yoga

The pancreas is a large gland tucked in behind your stomach. Not many people know what it actually does. But its two main jobs are, to help keep your blood sugar levels in a safe range and to make digestive juices that break down food in your intestines.

Pancreatitis happens when the digestive juices are activated before they leave your pancreas. This causes inflammation and swelling of your pancreas, pain in your abdomen, nausea and fever. Yoga may be a good way to reduce pain from chronic pancreatitis. A study showed that after three months of yoga people had less pain and needed fewer drugs.

Yoga is part physical, part mental and part spiritual. There are many different types of yoga and if you want to try it you should be able to find a class which suits your fitness level and exercise style. Classes usually run for an hour up to an hour and a half.

## Peppermint oil

It's the taste associated with Christmas and candy canes, peppermint is actually a cross between a spearmint and watermint. The peppermint plant is considered a pest in New Zealand, Australia and the Galapagos islands because it can grow on almost any surface. Peppermint oil might well be useful as a treatment for irritable bowel syndrome. After just one month, a study showed great improvements in three-quarters of people taking peppermint oil compared to people who did not.

Peppermint oil could, of course, be obtained by eating straight peppermint but it would be hard to consume enough to get any benefit from it. Supplements are therefore recommended if you want to try peppermint oil, but make sure you get the type that is intended for internal use only.

*There are many other medical conditions related to the stomach and bowels that it is thought peppermint might help, including indigestion, heartburn, nausea, vomiting, morning sickness, diarrhoea, cramps of the upper gastrointestinal tract and bile ducts.*

## Prebiotics

Prebiotics are the food that the good bacteria in your digestive system eat to stay healthy and effective. You yourself don't digest any of it, but it certainly keeps you digesting other food as efficiently as possible.

Prebiotics might be the answer if you are suffering from irritable bowel syndrome. A study showed that many symptoms of irritable bowel were improved after taking prebiotics for 3 months, including bloating and anxiety.

Stomach infections are never much fun, especially if you are a baby or the baby's parent. When prebiotics were added to infant formula, toddlers had fewer gut infections and needed fewer antibiotics than those who drank regular formula. It might be worth considering a prebiotic supplement if sore tummies are a regular complaint in your house.

## Psyllium

By swelling when it hits your intestines, psyllium helps you feel full and slows down your digestion. It is a type of soluble fibre that absorbs water and is added to some processed food as a thickener. Taking psyllium could be a good way to combat irritable bowel syndrome (IBS). An analysis of six studies showed that it was effective at reducing symptoms in people suffering from IBS.

Psyllium can be taken as a tablet, wafer or powder. Excess gas or stomach cramps sometimes occur as a side effect of taking psyllium, so make sure you talk to your doctor if you notice anything you are worried about. Make sure you drink plenty of water when taking psyllium.

*The average New Zealand adult eats 18-22 grams of fibre per day. This is lower than the recommended amount of 25g for women and 30g for men and some adults get less than half this amount.*

## Kiwifruit

The kiwifruit is actually native to China. It has had many names and its original Chinese name *yang tao* meaning 'sweet peach' was dropped when the fruit was imported to Europe as the Europeans decided it tasted far more like a gooseberry than a peach and it was commonly referred to as 'Chinese gooseberries'. When New Zealand farmers started growing it in 1962, they rechristened it kiwifruit to add to its market appeal.

Kiwifruit contains both soluble and insoluble fibre and along with the other valuable nutrients, the extra fibre can help if you are suffering from constipation.

Kiwifruit come in either green or a golden variety and one large kiwifruit contains 0.7 grams of soluble fibre and 1 gram of insoluble fibre. They can be eaten alone, in a fruit salad or atop a dessert.

## Synbiotics

A synbiotic is a supplement that contains both prebiotics *and* probiotics. In other words, both the good bacteria which are going to live in your gut and the food that they need to eat when they get there. Taking a synbiotic can improve your intestinal and digestive health.

A study showed improvements in stool frequency of people who took a synbiotic twice daily.

The typical dose for a synbiotic supplement is 1 to 10 billion active cells. That sounds like it would be a lot to eat, but don't worry - they're small and fit neatly into a capsule you can swallow or a powder that you can mix with a drink or yoghurt.

## Bovine Colostrum

In the same way mothers make breast milk to feed their babies, cows produce milk to feed their calves. In the very first few days after birth, the milk produced is called colostrum. This early milk is different to normal milk as it contains lots of immune boosting properties and nutrients. It has the ability to help your immune system fight an infection, or even kill off the infection itself.

If you have diarrhoea, you might want to consider using bovine colostrum to get it out of your system. Many studies have shown that it helps you get rid of symptoms of diarrhoea and may even stop you catching it in the first place if you consume colostrum on a regular basis.

Bovine colostrum is not drunk, but is instead turned into a tablet or powder before you take it. Many different variants are available. Differences occur because of what the cow was eating, how long after birth the milk was collected and how the product was processed.

*Some athletes use bovine colostrum to burn fat, build lean muscle, increase stamina and vitality, and improve athletic performance. It is not on the banned drug list of the International Olympic Committee.*

## Hypnosis

James Braid is called the father of hypnosis and coined the term hypnotism in 1841. He was preceded by mesmerists and magnetists but he thought that their ideas of telepathy and paranormal powers were absurd. Hypnosis allows the hypnotist to suggest ideas and thoughts to you while in a trance and has proven helpful in a few medical conditions.

One of these is chemotherapy-induced nausea and vomiting. An analysis of six studies showed that it can be very helpful, particularly in children.

Make sure you get someone with a lot of experience in the field to hypnotise you. You may need several sessions to see sustained results. We have no idea *how* it works, but for some people, for some conditions it can definitely be helpful (like when giving up smoking or conquering a fear of flying).

## Probiotics

Heavier than your heart and your brain, your body probably contains over one and a half kilos of these live bacteria. Considering how tiny they are, that is a very large number of organisms living inside of you, it has been estimated to be around 100 trillion! While probiotics live throughout your body, most are found in your intestines and digestive system helping you break down food and getting all the nutrients out. It makes sense that probiotics can be used for lots of issues with your stomach and bowels.

There is so much good research, for so many conditions that a case can be made that probiotics can help with almost any digestive system complaint. The conditions with the strongest evidence are:

### Diarrhoea

An average person will get diarrhoea once or twice a year. It is commonly caused by a virus in your intestines and can cause bloating, cramps, nausea and vomiting on top of the classic symptom.

Probiotic supplements are worth considering if you have diarrhoea. Studies which in total included over 8,000 people show that the length of your diarrhoea can be reduced by over 24 hours if you take probiotics.

### Antibiotic-Associated Diarrhoea

Antibiotics are taken to kill off bacteria that are causing problems, but they can also kill off good bacteria in your intestines. This can lead to diarrhoea. 40% of people who take antibiotics will suffer from diarrhoea. Taking probiotics can lower your risk of developing this problem.

36 studies with over 11,000 people in total showed that probiotics can lower your chances of getting diarrhoea when taking antibiotics by around 40%.

### Diarrhoea associated with HIV/AIDS.

HIV/AIDS can now be controlled to a large degree with modern medicines, but those medicines are not cheap and are not available in all parts of the world. Diarrhoea, flatulence and nausea are all common symptoms of HIV/AIDS that can be relieved with probiotics.

A small study of patients with these symptoms showed that almost everyone who took probiotics had no more diarrhoea, flatulence or nausea after just two days.

### Radiation-induced diarrhoea

Radiation therapy is often used as a way to kill off cancer cells. Unfortunately, diarrhoea is a common side effect of radiation that sometimes it is so bad that treatment cannot be continued. Taking probiotics can decrease your chance of developing diarrhoea during radiation treatment.

An analysis of ten studies showed a 56% drop in cases of diarrhoea amongst people receiving probiotics.

### Traveller's Diarrhoea

If you are travelling to Northern Africa, Latin America, the Middle East or Southeast Asia then there is a 50% chance that you will get traveller's diarrhoea.

*The risk of infection varies depending on the type of eating establishment visited, from fairly low risk in private homes to high risk in food from street vendors. The most common culprit is a bacteria called E.coli.*

Stress, jet lag and unfamiliar food can all make you more vulnerable to catching an infection. Luckily, probiotics might provide you with a solution.

Studies involving over 4,500 people show that taking probiotics during your trip can decrease your risk of diarrhoea by around 85%.

### Constipation

After all this talk of diarrhoea it seems strange that the same thing could work for constipation, but this does seem to be the case. Constipation is so common that at any point in time 2% of all people are suffering from constipation. It can be caused by not getting enough water or fibre, stress, change in routines or lack of exercise.

An analysis of five studies showed that probiotics can help to increase your number of bowel movements if you have constipation.

### Stomach Problems associated with Chronic Stress

Death of a family member, work, exams or relationship problems can all cause stress. For some people, if this stress is unrelenting it can lead to chronic stress. Chronic stress can cause abdominal pain, nausea and vomiting among other physical, psychological and sleep problems and is very bad for your health. Taking a probiotic can relieve many of the digestive related issues of chronic stress.

### Irritable bowel syndrome (IBS)

Nobody really knows what causes IBS despite the fact that one in five adults suffer from one or more of its symptoms at some time in their lives.

Cramps, pain, bloating, excess gas and fluctuation between diarrhoea and constipation are some signs that you could have IBS. Probiotics might help improve some of the symptoms.

20 small studies show that on average you have around a 25% chance of improvement by taking probiotics.

**Inflammatory Bowel Disease**

Crohn's disease and ulcerative colitis are both autoimmune diseases that cause similar symptoms in your digestive system. Abdominal pain, vomiting, diarrhoea, bleeding and weight loss are some of the nasty things sufferers have to deal with. They are much more serious diseases than IBS, which some people confuse them for.

These diseases sometimes go into remission. Taking probiotics might be effective for helping a person stay in this remission phase.

> *In medicine, remission means the disappearance of the signs and symptoms of a disease. This remission can be temporary or permanent.*

Studies of both Crohn's and ulcerative colitis show improvements in the length of remission when probiotics were added to their diet.

***Helicobacter Pylori*** **Infection**

Two thirds of people have this strain of bacteria in their bodies, but in most cases they aren't doing any damage. When they do, they eat through your stomach lining and can cause gastritis or ulcers. Taking a probiotic supplement could help treat a *Helicobacter pylori* infection.

An analysis of 10 studies involving nearly 1,500 people showed that probiotics could help kill off the nasty bacteria and reduce the side effects of other medications that may be taken to help eradicate it.

CHAPTER 08

# Brain and nervous system

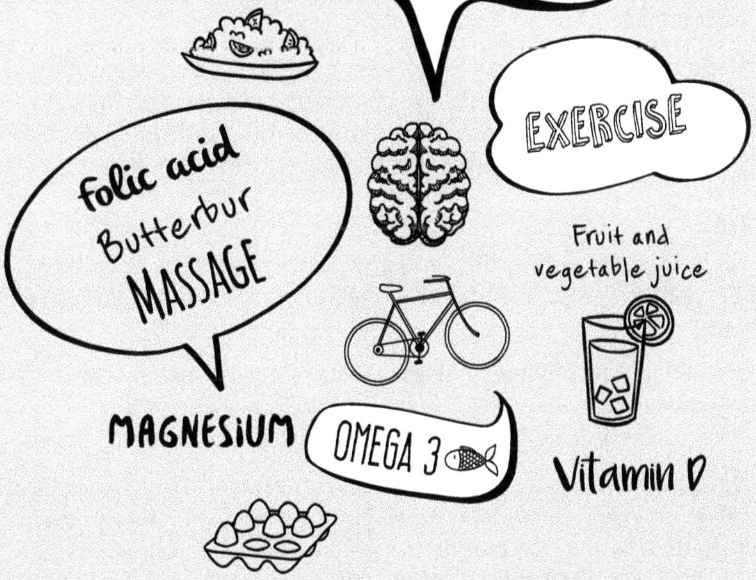

It's probably the most important organ in making you who you are and without it you wouldn't be able to read this sentence, turn the next page or even know that you are holding a book. Its importance is illustrated by the fact that your brain uses 20% of the oxygen you breathe in, despite making up only 2% of your total body weight. Around half of the genetic information in your DNA is instructions on how to keep your brain working, with the other 98% of your body having to share the rest.

You think over 70,000 thoughts a day and those are only the ones that you are aware of. So much of what your brain does, estimated to be around 90%, is background work, keeping your body working. But what happens when your brain starts to break down?

Being such a complex machine, it's not surprising that there are so many ways that it can go wrong. As life expectancy grows, so does the likelihood of your brain malfunctioning. Dementia, one of the most well-known and heart-wrenching ways the brain can stop working properly affects about one in ten people over the age of 65.

In this chapter, natural remedies for Alzheimer's disease and dementia, multiple sclerosis, epilepsy, ADHD and migraines are discussed. Ways to improve your brain's performance in memory, learning and speed are also covered.

## Omega-3

We've known about how they help you grow since the 1930s but only in the last 30 years have many of the other health benefits of omega-3 been discovered.

For people with mild Alzheimer's disease, a daily dose of fish oil can help slow down the disease. It can keep your brain working better for longer. Unfortunately, it probably won't help people with more advanced Alzheimer's.

A diet high in omega-3 can help improve your learning abilities and brain speed. A study of over 2,000 elderly Norwegians showed that eating 75 grams of fish a day gave them a huge advantage in test situations compared to people who ate no fish.

Toddler's brains are learning so much that their brains are rewiring constantly in order to keep up. There are some conflicting research papers when it comes to whether omega-3 can help young developing brains, but one impressive study found that four year olds who were given an omega-3 supplement used more words and had better listening skills that those who were not.

## Vitamin D

The definition of a vitamin includes that it cannot be made in your body and you can only get it through the food that you eat. This makes vitamin D's name a lie! You can make vitamin D when you are out in the sun, using your skin. Most adults make around 10% of their vitamin D this way.

Not getting enough vitamin D can slow down your brain. In a study of people aged over 65, those with the lowest amounts of vitamin D were more than two times more likely to suffer from certain types of brain impairments such as dementia.

*Dementia is a term that means 'a chronic or persistent disorder of the mental processes caused by brain disease or injury and marked by memory disorders, personality changes, and impaired reasoning.'*

Increasing your vitamin D levels can also lower your risk of getting multiple sclerosis. This is an autoimmune disease that disrupts your nervous system, making it more difficult for you to send messages around your body. Getting lots of vitamin D while under the age of 20 is strongly associated with stopping its development.

## Exercise

This is one treatment that has been around as long as us, but our early ancestors probably didn't see it that way. To them, exercises such as running, climbing, and swimming were simply a way to stay alive. We now know that regular exercise is not just good for your overall health, but can help keep your brain alive.

A study of 1,700 people showed that exercising at least three times per week lowered their risk of having dementia or Alzheimer's disease.

It is important not to over-do it, your fitness regime should be slowly increased, and there are plenty of specialists out there wanting to help you. A gym membership could be something you consider, the group classes which they offer can be a great way to meet new people and many gyms offer a free consultation with a personal trainer when you join. However, getting enough exercise can be as simple as walking the dog, playing with the kids or any activity that gets your heart pumping and gets you off the couch.

## Fruit and Vegetable Juice

Natural smoothies may be the latest healthy eating trend, but it's one that can have big health benefits. Fruit and vegetable juices have lots of nutrients in them, including ones that will protect your brain and nervous system from damage.

One study found that having three or more servings of fruit and vegetable juices a week could lower your risk of getting Alzheimer's by 80%! The study showed that the more you consume, the lower the risk.

You only have to look up 'fruit and vegetable smoothie recipes' to find hundreds of different recipes you will want to try. Dark coloured fruit like cranberries and blueberries are high in the nutrients you are after. Green leafy vegetables can also make an interesting addition to your juices.

## Folic Acid

This B vitamin is most commonly known for being taken as a prenatal supplement by expectant mothers to help stop birth defects in babies.

*There are eight B-group vitamins and they are essential for various functions within the body. Dietary supplements containing all eight are referred to as a vitamin B complex.*

It is also an important part of making the red blood cells which carry oxygen around in your blood. Your body needs folic acid for many other reasons as well and one of those is to help your brain work properly. Taking folic acid can improve your memory and speed up how quickly your brain will react to new information.

Your body cannot make folic acid, this means it has to be taken in from the food you eat, or from a supplement. It naturally occurs in leafy green vegetables, fruit and dried beans. Food can be fortified with it, meaning that it is added to the food during the manufacturing process.

## Yoga

The full name for the type of yoga which is commonly practiced in the Western world is Hatha Yoga. Hindu legend says that Hatha Yoga was created by the god Shiva on a deserted island. He was watched by a sneaky fish called Matsyendranath, who went on to share Shiva's secret yoga with the rest of the world. Practicing yoga morning and evening can potentially lower the number of seizures people with epilepsy experience.

A study showed that after 12 months of regular yoga, epilepsy sufferers reported that they had half the number of seizures they had before they started doing yoga.

Classes should be easy to find in your area. Once you have mastered the basics, you can continue practicing the mindfulness, breathing and poses that all make up an essential part of yoga by yourself.

## Pine Bark and Antioxidants

Migraines affect about 15% of people. Migraine attacks can include strong headaches, nausea and visual disturbances, such as rippling of your sight. They can last a few hours, or several days. Pycnogenol and other supplements high in antioxidants may lower the number of migraine attacks you have, as well as making them less painful when they do happen.

Many healthy organic food is naturally high in antioxidants. Try adding a handful of berries to your morning cereal, a stir-fry of colourful vegetables with your dinner, or a handful of nuts as an evening snack. If you choose to take a supplement, Pycnogenol is a good choice. Also look out for vitamins C and E, as these are well known antioxidant vitamins.

## Osteopathy

This manual therapy has only been around since 1874 when Andrew Still of Kansas linked bone structure to the functioning of your body. Osteopaths manipulate your bones and ligaments to help you unwind and stretch.

A study showed that osteopathy could help lower the number of headaches that people experience. Those who saw an osteopath once a week in this research reported that they had fewer headaches than before they began the treatment.

Make sure you visit a registered osteopath, as not doing so may cause more harm than good! Ask them to focus on your pelvis, cranium and spine (the areas worked on in the study) as a good starting point for your treatment. Osteopathy is designed to not just relieve your symptoms, but also to benefit your whole body.

## Massage

Records from ancient civilisations including China, Egypt and Rome have mentioned massage as early as 2,700 B.C. The tomb of Akmanthor (also known as 'The Tomb of the Physician') shows early Egyptian paintings of men receiving hand and feet massages from their servants. Our ancestors must have been onto something, as massage is used now not just for relaxation, but also for health treatments.

Massage therapy can potentially reduce the number of migraine attacks that sufferers have, improve quality of sleep, reduce stress and anxiety and leave you feeling better able to cope with daily life.

Massage typically includes pressure and movement on your soft tissues such as muscles, tendons and ligaments. Treatments designed especially for migraines use the trigger points on your back, shoulders, head, and neck to relieve muscle spasms and pain.

### B Vitamins

Parkinson's disease is named after James Parkinson who wrote the first detailed description of the disease in 1817. A high intake of vitamin B6 can potentially lower your risk of developing Parkinson's as you grow older.

B6 is important in sending messages across the brain and in protecting nerve cells from damage and a study showed that people who had a high intake of vitamin B6 were 30% less likely to get Parkinson's disease.

B6 can be found in liver, kidney, chicken and fish. Vegetarian sources include legumes such as beans and lentils which can be easily added to a stew or casserole. Various Vitamin B supplements are also available and as other B vitamins help with absorption taking a B complex is not a bad idea.

### Omega-3 and Omega-6

Not to be lumped together, omega-6 has a different function from omega-3. It is made in your body while you exercise and helps you grow and repair cells. Both omega-3 and omega-6 fatty acids may help to reduce symptoms of ADHD in children and teenagers.

Studies found that there is more likely to be a positive response from extra omega oils if the symptom was difficulty concentrating. It also seems to have a greater effect on boys rather than girls and also in people with autistic symptoms. If you or your children fit into any of these categories, increasing omega-3 and omega-6 levels may be worth trying.

You can raise your fatty acid levels by simply changing up the food you eat. Omega-3 oils are mainly found in oily fish or olive oil, while omega-6 levels are high in sunflower and canola oil. Nuts are also a great source of omega-6 that is easy to nibble on during the day. Supplemental versions are also available for both, with fish oils being higher in omega-3 with flaxseed oil being higher in omega-6.

### Meditation

Taken from the Latin meaning '*to think or ponder*' meditation has been associated with many religions and beliefs in the past. It is used to help you relax and people who practice it often report a benefit in terms of having more kindness and empathy through this quiet reflection. Children with

ADHD may benefit from meditation to help relieve stress, anxiety and other related symptoms.

> *ADHD is the short name for Attention-deficit/hyperactivity disorder. This is a brain disorder characterized by some or all of inattention, hyperactivity and impulsivity which can interfere with functioning or development.*

A study showed that students who meditated twice a day, for only 10 minutes each time, behaved better than those who did not.

The great thing about meditation is that it will not interfere with any medications or behavioural treatments. It may even make them more effective, as you will hopefully be more relaxed and responsive to them.

## Ginkgo Biloba

Extracts from this tree have been used in traditional Chinese medicine for thousands of years. With fossils showing us they have survived relatively unchanged for 270 million years, they are an extremely tough tree. Six ginkgo trees were growing 2 kilometres from the site where the Hiroshima bomb was dropped in 1945 and they are still standing today.

Gingko may be helpful for many health conditions. Over 50 studies have shown it may be effective for preventing and slowing Alzheimer's disease. It improves blood flow, boosts the immune system and works as an antioxidant.

Ginkgo biloba extract can be taken as a supplement in capsule or tablet form and the dose is around 120mg per day.

## Vitamin E

Vitamin E has the scientific name *tocopherol* which means '*to have children*', as increasing fertility was the first known medical use of the vitamin. In addition to helping you have children, vitamin E is also important in making the cells which carry oxygen around your body and helping you build muscles.

It works as an antioxidant, which means it may help in slowing the damage that Alzheimer's disease does to your body. Studies have shown that it may keep your brain working properly for longer, giving you a better quality of life.

Kiwifruit is a great source of vitamin E. Cooking your food in canola or sunflower oil, enjoying a handful of nuts, or making a leafy green salad for lunch are all excellent ways to increase how much vitamin E you are eating. Vitamin E can also be taken as a supplement, you will want around 400-800IU (international units) per day.

### Magnesium

It helps to keep your blood vessels nice and relaxed, which means magnesium helps keep you nice and healthy. Migraines may be triggered by your brain not getting enough oxygen from your blood. Keeping the blood flowing by making sure you get enough magnesium may help with migraine symptoms.

Studies have shown that taking magnesium while you have a migraine can lower the pain, in some cases making it disappear altogether. Taking it regularly may also mean you have fewer migraines.

Choosing whole grain food instead of their white counterparts can be an easy way to boost the magnesium in your diet. Nuts, beans and seeds are all great sources of magnesium as well. The mineral can also be taken as a supplement and is usually part of any good multivitamin.

### Butterbur

Flowering in winter and spring, butterbur is a member of the sunflower family that likes to grow in moist places such as riverbanks and marshes. It has been used as a natural remedy for almost 2,000 years and in the Middle Ages was thought to be a cure for the plague.

Butterbur can be used as a treatment for migraines, as it helps reduce swelling and calms muscle spasms. Studies show that taking a butterbur extract regularly can potentially halve the number of migraines you get per month.

*Note that we use words like potentially and may quite often....the truth is that not every therapy, or even medicine, works for everyone and so it's often a case of try and see.*

Butterbur can be taken as a supplement. It is important to make sure you buy a reputable brand, as butterbur that has not been properly processed can contain compounds that may damage your liver.

## Feverfew

Even though its name means '*fever cure*' the flower is not at all useful when you have a fever. Ancient Greeks used feverfew to help with headaches and evidence from modern medicine shows they might have been onto something.

Taking feverfew can reduce pain from migraines and cause you to have less migraine headaches overall. Studies show that feverfew can reduce many of the common migraine symptoms including nausea and light sensitivity, not just headache pain.

Feverfew can be taken as an extract, tablet or capsule. Be wary of interactions with medications that thin your blood, such as warfarin and let doctors know that you are using it if you are going to have surgery.

## Riboflavin

Also known as vitamin B2, riboflavin is an essential building block used to make skin, blood cells and other parts of your body. Not getting enough riboflavin can result in a sore mouth, eyes and a low mood. Riboflavin can be used to treat migraines. It 'revs up' your mitochondria so they produce more energy and it is thought that this extra energy can relieve migraine pain or even stop them happening in the first place.

*Mitochondria are tiny organelles inside cells that are involved in releasing energy from food. This process is known, confusingly, as cellular respiration.*

Many studies link taking riboflavin to suffering from fewer migraine headaches.

Animal products like milk, cheese and eggs have lots of riboflavin in them. Throwing some beans or lentils into a stew or bolognese is also an easy way to increase the amount you're eating. Supplements can be taken as another option.

## Coenzyme Q10

Coenzyme Q10, or CoQ10, or simply just Q10, increases the oxygen supply to your heart, making it work more efficiently. They also help your mitochondria, the energy factories of your cells, to make as much energy as possible. Making sure you have enough CoQ10 might reduce the number of migraines you have.

A three month long study showed that taking CoQ10 extract could lower the number of days you got a migraine and reduce the related nausea, which can be just as bad as the headache.

Your body can make CoQ10 on its own, but you might need a little extra to get the migraine-relieving benefits. Some of the best food to eat is chicken, beef, fish and oranges. You can also take supplements to boost your intake, look for around 50 - 150 mg of Coenzyme Q10 per day.

# CHAPTER 09
# Mental Health

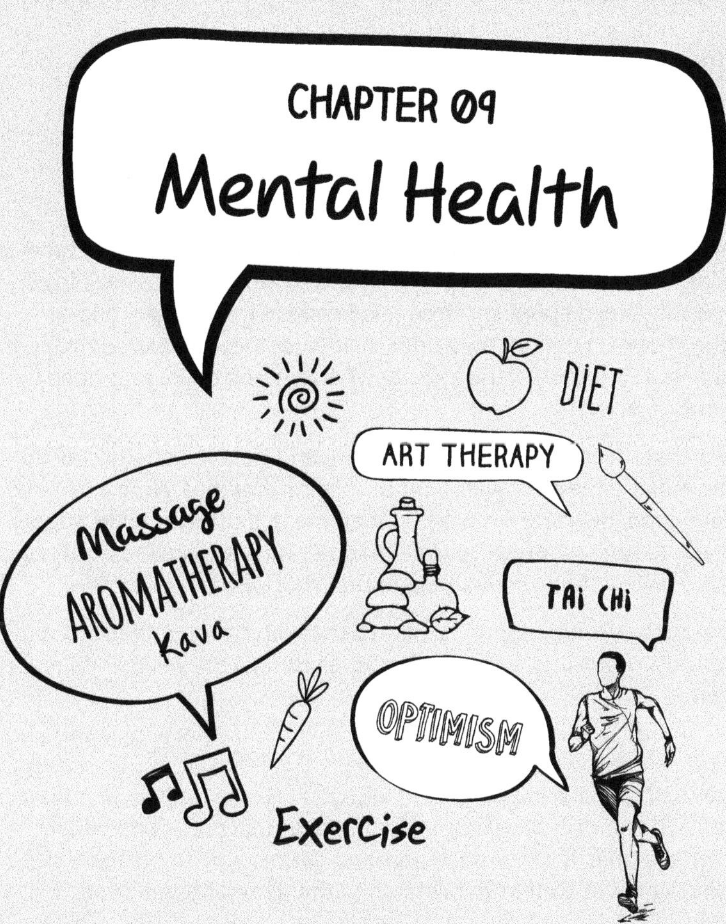

Just like any other organ in your body, your brain can have problems. Two of the most common mental health issues are depression and anxiety. One in four people will experience depression at some point in their life and women are twice as likely to suffer from depression as men. If one of your parents had a mental health problem, you are three times more likely to get the same thing than the average person.

It's not just all in your mind either; anxiety and depression can affect the health of your whole body. Depressed people suffer more colds each year than normal and having anxiety can make you think a smell is worse than it really is!

Many people who have a mental illness don't get the help they need. It is estimated that 80% of people with depression are not receiving any type of treatment. This can be because they find it hard to admit that something's wrong or that they need support. Often it is because they simply do not know that they have an illness, they think that what they are experiencing is normal. You might not understand exactly what is going on in your head and this can be very scary.

Doctors think that mental illnesses like anxiety and depression are caused by your brain making the wrong amount of mood hormones. Hormones that make you feel good, like serotonin and dopamine, are often in short supply. Treatments aim to not just make you feel happier and less anxious, but also to regulate the levels of hormones your brain produces.

This chapter looks at some natural remedies that can boost your mood and relieve symptoms of anxiety and depression, as well as a few other common mental illnesses.

## Massage

Used for over 5,000 years, massage can help you relax as well as providing health benefits. It can decrease levels of anxiety and depression in many situations. For example, it can reduce prenatal depression, depression in children/adolescents as well as depression in the general population.

An analysis of 37 studies found a large reduction in low mood symptoms including anger and anxiety when people had massage therapy. Levels of dopamine and serotonin increased, while cortisol levels went down.

*Cortisol is commonly known as the 'stress hormone,' as it influences, regulates or modulates many of the changes that occur in the body in response to stress.*

There are a variety of forms of massage and you are bound to be able to find one that suits you. Swedish massage is the most common type. Specialised massages include back massage, pregnancy massage, and sports massage. All massages involve pressure, rubbing and kneading of muscles and other soft tissue in your body.

### Meditation

Closing your eyes shuts off one of your senses and allows you to concentrate more easily. Some people close their eyes when trying to solve a problem or recall a forgotten fact. When you are meditating the aim is to shut off all information from the outside world.

Meditation has proven to be very effective at reducing symptoms of depression and other mental health disorders like anxiety, phobias and obsessive-compulsive disorder (OCD). It can be used alone or alongside standard medical therapies such as psychotherapy or medications.

Transcendental meditation, mindfulness meditation and visualisation are all types of meditation you might like to try. Attending a class or learning from a medical professional is a great way to start. Techniques can then be practiced at home. Apps for your smartphone are also now available that talk you through some basic meditation practices.

### Biofeedback

Skull caps full of sensors to monitor your brainwaves may seem like a science fiction concept but being able to see your body's responses as they happen can be game-changing for some mental health issues. Biofeedback, or neurofeedback, involves hooking yourself up to a computer that allows you to see your heart rate, blood pressure, tension and brain processes as they change. It allows you to see how different thoughts affect your body. Choosing thoughts that benefit your body is easier when you can see which thoughts are useful. It is also a great way to learn relaxation techniques.

This therapy may help people with depression, anxiety and other mental illnesses to re-train their brain into a healthier way of thinking. The process requires training and practice of certain patterns of thinking. Over time your brain remembers and automatically works this way, with no need for ongoing treatment or medications.

### Tai Chi

The full name of Tai Chi, *t'ai chi ch'uan*, translates as '*the first boxing*'. There are five major styles of Tai Chi, that all evolved from each other between the 18th and 19th centuries. Each style is named after the family who invented it. In every style, movements are slow, graceful and deliberate and breathing is rhythmic and controlled.

This relaxes the mind and the body and is said to balance the forces of yin and yang. Practicing Tai Chi can lead to less tension in your body as well as decreasing depression, anger, and anxiety.

You can learn Tai Chi from a teacher at a local class. Check your community centre or nearby gyms to find one in your area.

## Aromatherapy

Ancient Romans used scent in perfumes, cosmetics and medicines and this tradition has been carried on until today. The idea of aromatherapy was first written about in 1937 by a French chemist, Rene-Maurice Gattefosse. Essential oils are extracted from flowers, leaves, seed or fruit rinds and they can be effective treatments for many conditions including depression and anxiety.

A study showed a 30% decrease in mental health symptoms and a better sense of well-being among people who used aromatherapy.

*It is not fully known how aromatherapy works, but the 'smell' receptors in your nose communicate with the parts of your brain that act as storehouses for emotions and memories. Some researchers think that the oil vapours stimulate these parts of your brain and influence physical, emotional and mental health.*

Oils can be inhaled or applied to the skin. To inhale the scents effectively, you release them over steaming hot water and breathe deeply. Applying oils directly to your body is typically done in one of two ways: you can either bathe in water that has had the oils added to it, or they can be massaged directly onto your skin.

## Exercise

Easy and free (apart from the running shoes), exercise is a great hobby to get into. When you aren't feeling great it can be hard to motivate yourself, but in the end it will be worth it. Participating in exercise programmes can help with depression, anxiety and general well-being as well as being great for your body.

An analysis that looked at the results of many studies (with a total of more than 6,500 participants) showed that the more exercise you did each week, the fewer symptoms of depression you had. Part of the benefit may be from having more exposure to sunlight and the resulting increase in vitamin D levels.

Walking is a great starting point for your exercise regime. It's free, easy, has a low risk of injury and can be done almost anywhere. Other tips for people just getting started is to have a routine and to keep a record of what you have achieved in order to stay motivated.

## Diet

Processed food is quick and easy to cook when you are stressed, but could actually be contributing to your mental anguish. Low levels of fresh fruit and vegetables can cause depression, or make an existing condition worse. If you are feeling low, taking a careful look at what you are putting in your body can be a useful first step.

Your brain is fuelled by your blood which is in turn fuelled by the food you eat. Surveys have shown that eating lots of fresh, organic food is linked to good mental health.

As well as aiming for your 5+ a day, you can improve your mood by eating fibre-rich food like wholegrain bread, proteins (especially oily fish) and avoiding food that has a lot of sugar in it. Caffeine and alcohol, while being a great initial boost, can also make you feel lousy in the long run.

## Optimism

In terms of your mental health, it's definitely better that the glass is half full. This idiom is often used to show different viewpoints of the same situation. A pessimist would say the glass is half empty, while an optimist would go for half full.

Optimism has been shown to decrease depression and even extend your life expectancy. A study of 7,000 students found that being optimistic can boost the immune system and improve mental health.

Your levels of optimism are not set in stone. When faced with a situation that you would normally see as negative, focus on the good outcomes that can come from it. If you make a mistake work out how you can learn from it, to improve the way you'd do things next time, and don't worry about it too much. Just as playing sports improves with practice, the more you work on your optimism the better you will become at focussing on the positives.

## Tryptophan/5-HTP

In 1989, a large outbreak of a pain syndrome was first linked to tryptophan supplements and so it was banned in many countries. After an investigation into the outbreak, it was found that the cause was a single Japanese manufacturer of tryptophan whose supplements contained impurities. When it was discovered that it was these impurities that caused the problems most bans were lifted.

When tryptophan reaches your bloodstream, it gets turned into 5-HTP. Not having enough of this in your body can increase your anxiety levels and means you don't make much serotonin. Studies have shown that taking a tryptophan or 5-HTP supplement can lower your anxiety response and improve depressive symptoms.

Supplements of 5-HTP are available. Side effects that you might experience and need to be wary of include nausea, diarrhoea and difficulty breathing.

## Kava

Growing in the western Pacific, kava is a plant whose roots have long been used for sedating and relaxing without disrupting your ability to think clearly. The active ingredients in kava are called kavalactones.

There is evidence that suggests that these can help you deal with social anxiety. Many studies have been done on kava. One analysis of 11 studies found it to be an effective treatment for anxiety, while a different analysis of six studies found that its beneficial effects were comparable to commonly prescribed anxiety medications.

Kava is typically used as an ingredient in drinks in countries where it grows. These beverages are a great source of supplementary kava. Capsules and tablets are also available for you to take but you should avoid driving after taking them.

*It is a rare side effect, but there are several dozen reports of people who have had severe liver toxicity after consuming kava. The risk is reduced by having smaller amounts and by having breaks from taking it.*

## Valerian

A herb with pretty white or pink flowers, its name comes from the Latin word *valere* which means to be healthy and strong. Hippocrates and Galen both described its use as a treatment for insomnia and it is often recommended for people who suffer from anxiety.

Many studies have shown that it can reduce the severity of anxiety in people with generalised anxiety disorders and cause stress levels to drop when people had valerian in their system. One of the authors of this book always takes valerian the night before her exams!

Available as a supplement, it comes in capsule, liquid or tea forms. Beware that it has earned itself the nickname 'stinky socks' as this is exactly what some forms can smell like.

*As it is a sedative you should not drive or operate machinery after taking valerian. It can also interact with other sedatives (such as alcohol) so they should not be consumed at the same time.*

## Yoga

Combining asanas (poses), pramayama (breathing) and dhyana (meditation), Yoga aims to benefit your body and your mind. It was pretty much unheard of in the west just over a century ago. In the mid-19th century Yoga began to get popular, when Indian philosophy and religion gained interest in Western countries. Yoga can help you to reduce stress and nervousness within your body. Hormones in your blood respond to your calmness and levels of stress hormones such as cortisol, prolactin and oxytocin levels can reduce after doing Yoga.

A study showed that Yoga reduced depression symptoms and lowered the chance of future depression.

Yoga can be learnt at a local community centre, gym or a Yoga studio. Each teacher will have a different style, so shop around a bit until you find one you like. Practicing at home between classes will help you see faster improvements in your mental health.

## Art Therapy

Since humans first gained the understanding of life beyond everyday survival, recording what happens has been an important part of our culture. Cave paintings and bone carvings are some of the first evidence of art, but it's likely that even before then art was created that simply did not stand the test of time.

The creativity and self-expression involved in making art can be healing and help you discover your feelings and emotions. Studies show that people with depression can really benefit from art therapy in particular.

It doesn't just have to be about drawing. Painting, sculpture or photography can all be used and it's not about your artistic abilities. Exploring repressed emotions and resolving personal conflicts is the aim of the game. Art therapy classes may be offered where you live, or just give it a try yourself.

## Music Therapy

Ancient Greeks believed that music could heal the body and mind, and soldiers returning from World War II were some of the first to be treated with music therapy to help with shock. Music stimulates your body and encourages it to release feel-good hormones that can improve your mood.

It can be used to treat depression, with studies showing that music therapy can improve both your thought processes and depressive symptoms.

You don't have to be musically talented to benefit from musical therapy. While playing an instrument or writing songs is very therapeutic and should be considered as an option, listening to music and talking about the meaning of songs can help you gain a better understanding of yourself. If music classes sound like your thing, pick an instrument and find a local teacher. Alternatively there are many teach yourself books and online videos for common instruments like the guitar or piano. Remember to consider your neighbours mental health before you buy that drum set.

## Dance and Movement Therapy

Dance is an important part of every culture. From ballet to Maori haka, dance has always been a way for people to express themselves. It may be an excellent hobby/treatment for people suffering from depression. It's not for everyone, but for some, it can help you connect with yourself and with others and can provide you with a constructive way of acting out your frustrations.

Many studies have found that it can be helpful. For example, a study of teenage dancers showed that the longer they remained part of a dance class, the happier and less depressed they became.

If you have difficulty opening up and speaking about yourself, then dance therapy could be a great option for you. It combines exercise with an outlet for personal expression. Dance classes are not just for kids, and there are many different genres and styles for you to choose from.

## Hypnotherapy

The Greek word *hypnos* means to sleep and while hypnosis doesn't actually put you to sleep you enter a trance-like state that you might not remember when you 'wake up'. Hypnotism may seem very new-age but hieroglyphics on the walls of Egyptian tombs suggest that it was used as long as 3,000 years ago. It can potentially relieve depression by teaching you coping strategies and healthier, more productive thought patterns.

There are three stages of hypnosis. The pre-suggestion phase is used to focus your mind and put you into a relaxed state. The suggestion phase questions our goals, motive and memories. The post-suggestion is where you practice the new behaviours and thinking patterns learned in the suggestion phase. Make sure you find a qualified hypnotist to take you through the process in order to get the benefits you want.

## B Vitamins

Back in the 1920s, doctors thought that anaemia and folate deficiency were the same disease. They know now that anaemia is caused by a lack of red blood cells. They also know that folic acid and the other closely related B vitamins could help your brain make chemicals like serotonin and dopamine.

If you suffer from depression, folic acid might increase the effectiveness of the prescribed medications. Studies have also showed that having higher levels of B vitamins means people are less likely to suffer from depression.

As with many other nutrients, those green leafy vegetables are great places to start looking for some extra B vitamins. Oranges, beets, turkey and soybeans are other options you could try. If you take a supplement, look for one with vitamins B1 and B3.

## Light Therapy

In 400 BC Hippocrates noticed that '*the changes in seasons produce disease.*' One of the diseases he might have been talking about is seasonal affective disorder, which is often, appropriately, shortened to SAD.

*SAD is more common in females, younger people, people who have blood relatives with SAD or another form of depression and people who live a long way north or south of the equator.*

If you suffer from this, you experience recurrent depression during the colder seasons. A lack of light exposure is one of the contributing factors to this common condition. As the days get shorter, your body's natural clock can get messed up. Light therapy is a solution to this problem. Light exposure at the right times of day can have a positive effect on your mood and decrease symptoms of depression.

There are some commercially available products like light boxes which produce bright, strong light. Your other option is of course to spend more time in the sunshine. This can be difficult sometimes when the weather's bad, but a sunrise walk, could really help your mood for the rest of the day.

## Chromium

While pure chromium is a shiny silver colour, the origin of its name *chroma,* is a Greek word meaning colours. This is because many of the compounds it forms when it mixes with other elements are brightly coloured.

Research shows that chromium might change your body's response to the hormone serotonin and this makes it a possible treatment for depression. Studies have found that it is particularly good for people with atypical depression; a type of depression that causes excessive sleeping and appetite, quick mood changes and makes you more sensitive to rejection.

Chromium can be found in food like mashed potatoes and breakfast muffins. Broccoli, bananas and green beans are great healthy sources of it as well. Supplements are also available but you only need a tiny amount.

## St John's Wort

This little flowering plant is named after St John the Baptist, because the sap of the plant was said to bleed red after he was beheaded. In the Northern hemisphere, the day it flowers often coincides with St John's Day on June 24th.

It is often recommended for people with depression and there are many studies that back up its effectiveness as a treatment. One analysis of 25 different studies said it was very effective at treating mild-to-moderate depression and resulted in a similar reduction of symptoms as conventional antidepressants.

St John's Wort is available as a supplement in capsule or cream form. Beware of side effects though, the most common ones being restlessness, anxiety, irritability, stomach upset, fatigue, dry mouth, dizziness and headache.

## SAMe

S-adenosyl-L-methionine is a bit of a mouthful to say, so it's commonly called SAMe (pronounced sammy). It's present in every cell in your body and helps to make many important hormones like serotonin and dopamine. Your liver is responsible for making SAMe, but sometimes it doesn't make enough.

If you have depression, there's a chance that you have low levels of SAMe. Studies show that taking SAMe can increase the levels of 'good-mood' hormones in your blood and relieve symptoms of depression.

Oral supplements of SAMe are available to try. Unlike some other natural products that can help with depression, SAMe has very few side effects.

## Omega-3

This oil really is a wonder-food. Many people do not get enough of it, and deficiency in omega-3 is estimated to be responsible for over 100,000 deaths each year. As well as helping with blood pressure, diabetes, pain and boosting your immune system, there is evidence that suggests people who suffer because of their mental health could be helped by omega-3.

It might help with depression, schizophrenia and bipolar disorder. A three month study showed improvements in levels of depression and stress of people who have previously self-harmed. Also a study of people with schizophrenia found it reduced their symptoms in many cases without any nasty side effects.

Oily fish is one of the best places to get this nutrient. Nutritionists recommend aiming to eat fish at least twice a week. Fish oil supplements are also available including cod liver oil (just like Mum forced on you).

# CHAPTER 10
# Bones and Joints

Vitamin B
Chondroitin
SPA THERAPY
CALCIUM
Glucosamine
SOY
SEAWEED
Omega-3

From the Greek *arthron*, arthritis simply means disease of the joints. Most of us assume it's just something that happens as you get older but arthritis can affect anyone, even young children. It does become more common as you get older though, affecting 1 in 250 children, 1 in 5 adults, and almost 1 in 2 people over the age of 65. There are two predominant types, osteoarthritis and rheumatoid arthritis.

You have squishy pads in all of your joints that stop your bones from rubbing painfully together. This is called cartilage and over time, the cartilage gets worn down from years of use. When the cartilage wears away so much that the bones come into contact, this can cause pain, stiffness in your joints and difficulty moving as you used to. This type of arthritis is called *osteoarthritis*. Injuries, joint abnormalities and genetic factors can make you more likely to get osteoarthritis. It occurs in many other species, including cats, dogs and in the oldest recorded case, a fossil was used to diagnose osteoarthritis in *Allosaurus fragilis*, a large species of dinosaur.

*Rheumatoid arthritis* is different and thankfully rarer. It is an autoimmune disease, meaning your own body is the one doing the damage. For some reason, your immune system sees the tissue at your joints as a threat and attacks it, causing swelling, stiffness and pain. Over time it weakens the bones of your joints, making them change shape and making it more difficult for you to move. It is not clear exactly where the word rheumatoid comes from: it may have been first used to say that the joint swelling looked similar to that seen in rheumatic fever. Another possibility is that it comes from the word *rhuma* meaning water, and refers to how wet weather can sometimes make the symptoms worse.

## Soy

Nicknamed the '*golden bean*' in 20th century America, the soybean is an edible bean grown worldwide. The Americans and Europeans ate lots of soybeans during WWII, as it is a great source of protein that could be grown and stored more easily than other sources such as meat. Eating lots of soy may make your bones stronger and less likely to break.

*Bones that become brittle and more fragile are responsible for around 9 million fractures worldwide every year. The National Osteoporosis Foundation estimated last year that more than 10 million U.S. adults over the age of 50 have thin bones.*

A study showed that women who ate more isoflavones (one of the most important ingredients in soybeans) had stronger bones compared to those who did not. The more soy that was eaten, the greater the effect.

Soy can be easily added to your diet. Soybeans can be bought fresh, tinned, dried or frozen and can be added to many meals. Roasted soybeans make a delicious snack. Or maybe you could try switching over to soy milk instead of dairy. Isoflavone supplements are also available.

### Calcium

Calcium is one of the most common metals in many mammal's bodies. It is used to build teeth, bones and shells. Unsurprisingly, getting plenty of calcium can strengthen your bones and make you less likely to suffer from a fracture or break. A study of over 1,400 women has shown that over a five year period, people who took a calcium supplement regularly had fewer broken bones than those who did not. The key is to take it regularly as the best results are obtained if you remember to take it every day.

You can also increase your calcium levels by making changes to the food you eat. Dairy products such as milk, yoghurt and cheese are obvious choices that have loads of calcium. Green leafy vegetables, such as kale and broccoli are also good choices. Fruit juice and cereal sometimes have added calcium in them as well.

### Vitamin B

There are 8 different types of B vitamins and they all do different things. Vitamin B1 turns sugar into energy, while vitamin B9 helps your body make red blood cells.

*The types of B vitamins are B1 (Thiamine) - B2 (Riboflavin) - B3 (Niacin/nicotinic acid) - B5 (Pantothenic acid) – B6 (Pyridoxine/Pyridoxal/Pyridoxamine) – B7 (Biotin) – B9 (Folic acid/Folate) – B12 (Methyl cobalamin).*

A study found that having lots of vitamin B6 and B12 in your body lowered your risk of bone loss, hip fracture and osteoporosis. Hip fractures are definitely something you want to avoid, up to a third of elderly people who get a hip fracture die within a year.

Vitamin B6 is found in meat and whole grains. Liver has especially high levels of it and luckily also of vitamin B12. B12 only occurs naturally in animal products, including kidney, fish and dairy products. Vitamin B supplements are also available, just make sure they contain the right type.

## Vitamin C

Sailors on the high seas used to get sick with an illness known as scurvy. Many remedies were tried, including cider, seawater, sulphuric acid and vinegar before a fellow named James Lind proved that citrus fruit was the best cure. At the time, they suspected it was because of the acidic taste of the fruit, but we now know that it is due to the high levels of vitamin C.

Vitamin C can help older men reduce their bone loss as it helps to form collagen, which makes the scaffolding of your bones. A study found that it only had this effect in men and not women, for reasons unknown.

Many types of fruit and vegetables contain lots of vitamin C, including kiwifruit, strawberries, lemons, cabbage, snow peas, grapefruit, zucchini and pineapple.

*Surprisingly, a 80g serving of Brussel sprouts contains four times more vitamin C than an orange.*

## Three lesser known natural products that can strengthen bones

With so many natural health remedies claiming to do so much, it can be hard for you to know what to take. A large study tested a number of the less well known natural products that are used for treating and preventing bone problems and concluded that three in particular were helpful; phytoestrogens, dehydroepiandrosterone (DHEA) and vitamin K2.

Phytoestrogens are estrogen-like hormones that are made by plants. They are thought to have numerous positive effects on your body and protect you from many diseases, particularly those related to bones. Phytoestrogens are made in most plants and are found in vegetables, fruit and other plant based food, but not in animal products.

DHEA is a substance made naturally in your body that later turns into estrogen and other important hormones. Increased levels of these hormones reportedly boost your immune system, slow down the effects of aging and maintain healthy bones.

Vitamin K2 has also been shown to help bones and works along with calcium and magnesium. The best source of vitamin K2 is from fermented food like cheese, soybeans (*natto*) and sauerkraut. If taking it by way of a supplement choose the natural form MK-7 (menaquinone-7) not the cheaper synthetic MK-4 (menaquinone-4).

## Pycnogenol

Pycnogenol comes from pine trees in Europe's largest forest. Found in southwestern France, it is a man-made forest made almost entirely of *Pinus pinaster*, or French Maritime Pine trees.

Pycnogenol supplements can reduce symptoms in people with mild to moderate osteoarthritis. A study showed that after three months people taking pycnogenol had less pain and needed less medication than people who were not taking it.

It can also potentially have lots of positive side effects for you and we have mentioned it several times in this book. It may also decrease your blood pressure, increase your awareness, learning ability and memory, and improve your skin and hair quality.

## Chondroitin

Chondroitin is a chemical that is found around your bone joints. It is a big part of the cartilage that stops your bones rubbing painfully against each other. It makes sense that chondroitin supplements have been shown in many studies to help people with osteoarthritis. It helps to lessen joint pain, swelling, stiffness and to make it easier for people with osteoarthritis to move around, while also slowing down joint damage.

It's not really something you can get enough of through your food, so it should be taken as a supplement. Be careful about taking it at the same time as blood thinning drugs though, as they can work together to make your blood dangerously thin.

## Massage Therapy

The word massage is thought to come from the Arabic word *massa*, meaning to touch and to feel. The most common type of massage is Swedish massage, although it is only in English and Dutch that it is called this. In other languages it is simply called '*classic massage*'.

It has been shown to help many people with osteoarthritis by increasing relaxation and lowering pain levels. A study showed that people receiving one-hour sessions of massage either once or twice a week reported less pain than those who did not.

It is important that you find a properly trained masseuse to do your massage, as otherwise you run the risk of damaging your body instead of helping it.

## Boswellia Serrata

Depending on your beliefs, a gift that was given to the baby Jesus could also help you with your arthritis. Extracts from *Boswellia serrata* were known in biblical times as frankincense. It has been known to have anti-inflammatory power for a long time, its first uses being in Ayurvedic medicine (the traditional medical system in India).

For people with osteoarthritis it can help reduce your joint swelling, improve blood flow to your joints, lessen your pain and help you get around. A six month study showed people who took *Boswellia serrata* found it easier to complete daily activities than those who did not.

It can be taken as a supplement, usually in the form of a resin extract.

### Spa Therapy

Radon baths were first used in Austria, long before anyone even knew what radon was. Naturally occurring springs are present in many parts of the world, particularly Europe and Asia. These spring waters can be helpful for people suffering from rheumatoid arthritis.

A study showed that people with arthritis who took radon baths reported they found daily living easier, were more mobile and even felt like they needed their arthritis medications less, compared to those people who took carbon dioxide baths.

> *While Radon has been linked to lung cancer this is in much higher levels than that experienced in bathing and the benefit of these very low doses of radiation outweighs the potential risk.*

Radon baths are not available in New Zealand. However Rotorua's hot pools are often filled with natural spring water and have been reported to have similar effects to radon baths in reducing arthritis symptoms.

### Seaweed

Seaweed bathing houses have been around since the early 20th century. People suffering from arthritis would go to the bathing house and sit in a spa or hot bath full of seaweed for the pain relief it provided.

Seaweed products can be helpful in reducing symptoms of arthritis as seaweed lowers high levels of acid in your body that can cause arthritis. For people with moderate to severe osteoarthritis, a study showed that seaweed supplements reduced pain and joint stiffness and made it easier to move around.

Some seaweed bathing houses are still open around the world. But if that doesn't appeal, seaweed supplements are available.

*Traditionally, Chinese people have used hot water extracts of seaweed in the treatment of cancer, Japanese people have used seaweed to treat thyroid diseases and the Romans used seaweed in the treatment of wounds, burns, and rashes.*

## Devil's Claw

Devil's claw is a plant that was named after the hooked spikes of its strange looking fruit. It is native to southern Africa where it has been a traditional medicine to ease pain and indigestion for many years. European colonists first brought the plant home to treat arthritis in the 1800s.

It can still be helpful for people suffering from osteoarthritis by lessening their symptoms. Studies have shown that taking it can lower the amount of pain you feel as well as how many traditional painkillers you need to take.

Devil's claw can be taken as an herb, liquid, or capsule. It can also be drunk as a tea.

## Tai Chi

Tai chi is a Chinese martial art whose name comes from the mandarin phrase *tàijí quán* which translates as '*supreme ultimate boxing*'. Rhythmic movements flow smoothly into one another, and tai chi training is regarded as a partly physical and partly spiritual experience.

Tai Chi can be used to reduce pain and improve overall health. Studies show that people with arthritis who practice tai chi often have fewer symptoms and have a more positive view of their health in general.

Tai chi classes are available in most major places. You can also find tai chi videos aimed specifically at people with arthritis online.

*At the time of writing, tai chi lessons are available in many parts of New Zealand sometimes funded by the Accident Compensation Corporation - see www.acc.co.nz for more information.*

## Omega-3

Omega-3 fatty acids can reduce inflammation. As rheumatoid arthritis is an autoimmune disease which causes inflammation, making sure you get plenty of omega-3 can lessen the symptoms associated with it.

Studies showed that people who had higher levels of omega-3 had less stiffness in their joints and less pain overall. This included fewer and shorter flare-ups, a common symptom of rheumatoid arthritis.

You can improve your intake of omega-3 by eating lots of oily fish like salmon and mackerel. Walnuts or flaxseeds can be added to your muesli for an omega-3 boost. If you do not eat much of this type of food, you may want to consider taking a supplement, especially as fish oil has lots of potential benefits as well as helping with arthritis.

## Glucosamine

Glucosamine is important for keeping your joints well-oiled and padded. It is an important part of the cartilage on the ends of your bones, delaying the break down that occurs with age.

Glucosamine can help with arthritis. Studies showed that taking a glucosamine supplement can help keep your cartilage healthy, as well as reducing pain and the other symptoms associated with arthritis. In some studies it was as effective as commonly prescribed drugs.

You normally cannot eat glucosamine in large enough amounts to be helpful. Supplements are available and they are often made from the shells of shrimp, lobster or crab or made in a laboratory.

## Omega-3 and Glucosamine

Both omega-3 and glucosamine have already been mentioned in this chapter, but it's worth noting that taking them together can be of extra benefit. The two substances work synergistically. That means that the combined effect of taking them together, is more than the benefit you would get from them individually.

Taking omega-3 makes glucosamine more effective, and vice versa. Glucosamine looks after your cartilage, while omega-3 stops the swelling around your joints.

As mentioned earlier, you can improve your omega-3s with different types of fish and other food, or with supplements. However glucosamine is best taken as a supplement to make sure you get enough for the full benefit.

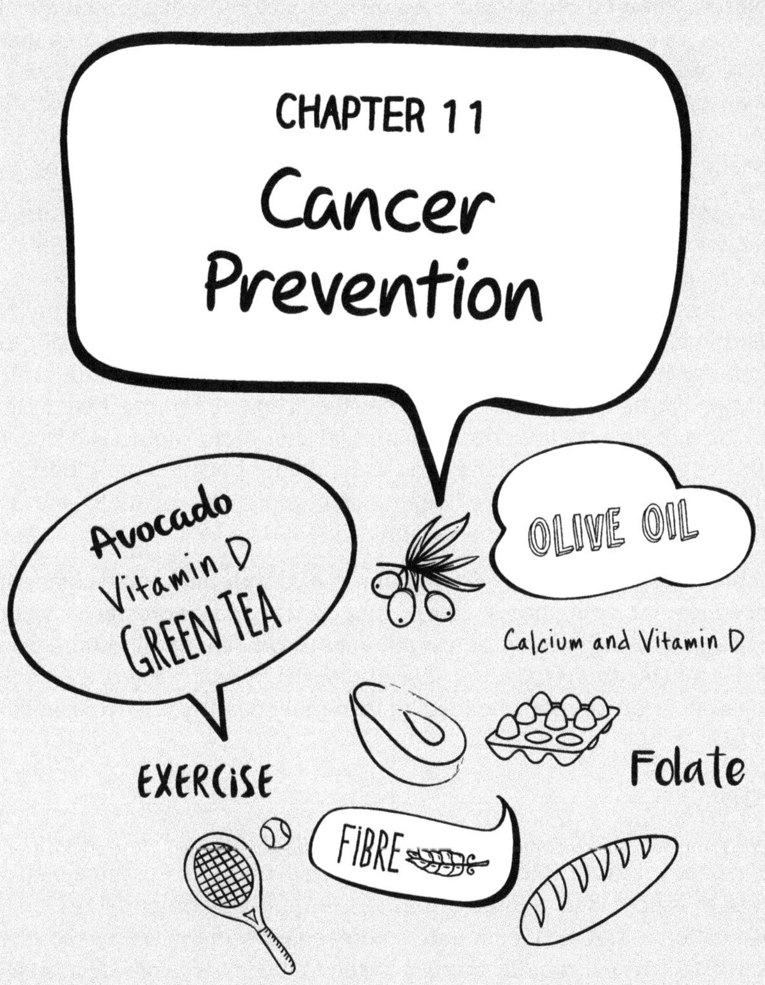
CHAPTER 11
Cancer Prevention
Avocado
Vitamin D
GREEN TEA
OLIVE OIL
Calcium and Vitamin D
Folate
EXERCISE
FIBRE

It is one of the biggest killers of our time and you have a 50% chance of getting some type of cancer during your life. Cancer causes an eighth of all deaths worldwide and is responsible for more deaths than AIDS, tuberculosis and malaria combined. Smoking causes 90% of all lung cancers. Men are slightly more likely to get lung cancer than women, because more men than women smoke. For women, the most common cancer risk is breast cancer. Breast cancer is not just a women's disease though and 1% of breast cancer sufferers are male. In total there are over 100 types of cancer that doctors know about and they can affect any part of your body.

Cancer happens when normal cell division in your body gets out of control. Cells divide to make new cells all the time. These new cells are used to fix wounds, replace dying cells and as part of normal growth in parts of the body such as the hair and fingernails. If something goes wrong, cells can begin to divide more than they should. A tumour is a group of cells that has grown rapidly in a place they shouldn't. Sometimes tumours are quite safe and just need to be cut out, but sometimes they can't be removed because they are tangled up with important organs like your brain. Metastasis is when cancerous cells from the tumour spread around your body in your blood. This can cause the cancer to take hold in one or more new locations and is generally really bad news for your health.

This chapter looks at ways to reduce your risk of developing some common types of cancer including breast cancer, lung cancer and colorectal (bowel) cancer, using natural remedies and supplements. Do bear in mind though that we are talking about reducing your risk, not eliminating the risk entirely. Unfortunately, even people who lead an incredibly healthy lifestyle can still get cancer.

## Olive Oil

The International Olive Council controls the quality of over 95% of olive oil and other olive products sold worldwide. Men from northern Europe are at higher risk of cancer than men from southern Europe. One potential reason for this observation is that olive oil is eaten more regularly in the warmer southern regions, which is why it is quite strongly linked to the lower levels of cancer.

A study of 180 European males showed that eating olive oil every day reduced the amount of certain chemicals in the blood which are associated with a higher risk of cancer.

*The main type of fat found in all kinds of olive oil is monounsaturated fatty acids (MUFAs). We do need some fat in our diet and MUFAs are considered to be a healthy dietary fat.*

You can use olive oil as a dressing or in cooking. It can also just be taken as is, but mixing it with a strong flavoured juice can make it easier for you to swallow.

## Avocado

The avocado is thought to come from Mexico and its name resembles the Spanish word *abogado* meaning advocate or lawyer. Including avocado in your diet may help to prevent cancer as it contains lots of the phytochemicals known to reduce cancer risk. As well as containing vitamins A, B6, C, D and E, they are high in antioxidants that stop cell damage.

On an avocado, the darker the flesh, the more nutrients that area of the fruit contains. The sections closest to the skin are the darkest green and the best way to access them is often by peeling the skin off with your fingers instead of scooping out the flesh.

> *Yes an avocado is a fruit, not a vegetable. In fact it is specifically, a single-seeded berry.*

In many countries avocado is typically eaten as a savoury food but in the Philippines and Brazil it is commonly added to sweet dishes. Avocado milkshakes and ice-creams are some recipes you could branch out and try.

## Omega-3

Oily fish contain up to 30% oil in their fillets but don't worry, this oil it good for you. It contains omega-3, an unsaturated fatty acid whose health benefits have been researched since the 1930s.

Consuming omega-3 fatty acids regularly might lower your risk of developing colorectal (bowel) cancer. A 22 year study showed that men who ate fish five times a week (or regularly took a fish oil supplement) lowered their chance of having colorectal cancer by 40%.

Tuna, salmon, mackerel and trout are all classified as oily or oily fish. Whitefish is the name for fish that are not high in oil content. These whitefish still contain all the same nutrients, just in much lower levels.

## Vitamin D

You are at risk of having low vitamin D if you have dark skin, don't get outdoors in the sun often or have digestive issues that stop you absorbing fat properly. Being at risk of low vitamin D also increases the risk you have of developing colorectal cancer.

An analysis of five studies showed that the less vitamin D you have the more likely it is you will get this type of cancer. Getting the right amount of vitamin D can potentially lower your risk by 50%.

*Around one third of New Zealanders have low levels of vitamin D. As we cover up more from the sun we are reducing our vitamin D levels.*

Most of your vitamin D comes from being in the sun. Your skin has to be in direct sunlight to make vitamin D and wearing sunscreen will reduce the amount of vitamin D you make. Of course, sunscreen is very important to ensure you don't get a different type of cancer. So try to ensure you get a few minutes of direct sunlight every day, but don't stay too long to avoid getting burned. It's a fine balance.

## Calcium

Some animals get a taste for calcium and will deliberately seek out calcium-rich rocks to lick. In humans the taste is not particularly pleasant and opinion varies remarkably between each person. When you eat calcium, you could think it tastes salty, sour or even soothing.

Taking a calcium supplement may reduce your risk of colorectal cancer and other cancers associated with your digestive system. A huge study of over 490,000 people showed that increasing calcium intake reduced the chance of getting colorectal cancer by 29%.

While calcium licks are popular with some animals, there are better tasting options for your diet that contain lots of calcium. Dairy products are an obvious choice, with milk, yoghurt and cheese all adding calcium to your diet. Leafy green vegetables also contain a surprising amount, or try a supplement to ensure a regular dosage.

## Calcium and Vitamin D

Both of these have just been mentioned, but increasing your calcium and vitamin D levels *together* will likely further protect women against breast cancer. We know that they work together to build strong bones and it also seems they work together to protect premenopausal women against breast cancer.

A ten year study following 32,000 women found a lower risk of breast cancer in women with higher levels of calcium and vitamin D.

Cheese lovers will be pleased to hear that it is one food that contains high levels of both vitamin D and of calcium. While most vitamin D comes from the sun, food that will increase your levels also include oily fish, eggs and liver.

## Ginseng

The Chinese name for ginseng is *renshen*. This can be translated as 'plant root person' and comes from the fact that the root can look remarkably like a small person with arms and legs. Taking a regular supplement of ginseng may reduce your risk of developing breast cancer.

Almost 1,500 people with breast cancer participated in a study that showed people who took ginseng had better quality of life, reduced risk of death and a lower chance of the breast cancer recurring.

You cannot get ginseng naturally from any common food and the root itself is hard to come by in most places. Your best bet for increasing your ginseng intake is to get yourself a supplement from a well-respected company; but beware: ginseng is an expensive root and some brands may not be entirely honest about how much is in each dose.

*Ginseng is increasingly being grown commercially in New Zealand, it grows particularly well in the Bay of Plenty because of the climate and free-draining volcanic soil.*

## Fibre

Humans lack the chemicals needed to break down and absorb fibre into our bodies. Animals like cows and horses have this chemical and this allows them to get nutrients from their grass and hay-based diets. However, you can use fibre to slow down your digestion and absorb the things you need from other food.

By increasing their fibre intake, pre-menopausal woman may be protected from breast cancer. A study showed that the higher the dose, the lower the chance. The highest dosage saw a 52% reduction in the risk of breast cancer.

It's not hard to find tasty food loaded with fibre. Choose natural, organic options as often the manufacturing process can remove fibre. Brown, grainy bread, wholemeal rice and pasta, beans, fruit and vegetables are great places to start if you are looking to increase your fibre.

## Folate

Folate and folic acid (vitamin B9) comes from the Latin word *folium* which means leaf. This is because green leafy vegetables are one of the best sources of it.

In post-menopausal women, increased folate intake lowered the chance of developing breast cancer. A study of over 11,000 women showed that high folate levels can lower the risk by 44%.

You cannot make your own folic acid, you have to get it from the food you eat. Spinach, asparagus, broccoli and parsley are all excellent plant based foods that can increase the amount of folic acid in your body. Citrus fruit and fruit juice is another easy way to get more of this vitamin.

## Green Tea

When green tea is brewed in the classic way, it is more than 99% water and only contains one calorie per 100ml. The length and temperature at which the tea is brewed depends on the quality of the tea leaves. High quality teas are brewed in cooler water for shorter periods, as the flavours escape more readily.

Drinking green tea regularly might reduce your chance of getting breast cancer. A study of 6,000 women showed that drinking green tea at least twice per week lowered their risk by around 12%.

Green tea can be drunk the same way you would drink black tea or coffee. It can be drunk with food or between meals. It can also calm and relax you before bed, but make sure you choose a decaffeinated tea to drink in the evenings, as green tea contains more caffeine than regular black tea.

## Exercise

Exercise is commonly recommended for health reasons of course. But one lesser known benefit is cancer prevention.

It can reduce the risk of lung cancer in smokers, of breast cancer in postmenopausal women and of bowel cancer in everyone. One study showed that at least four hours of exercise a week reduces your chances of getting cancer.

You can see the greatest benefits by doing a high-energy 'vigorous' exercise session at least twice a week, or a more gentle, 'moderate' exercise session at least four times a week. Vigorous activities include running, swimming and active team sports, while golf, walking and gardening are seen as moderate exercise activities.

# CHAPTER 12
# Women's Health

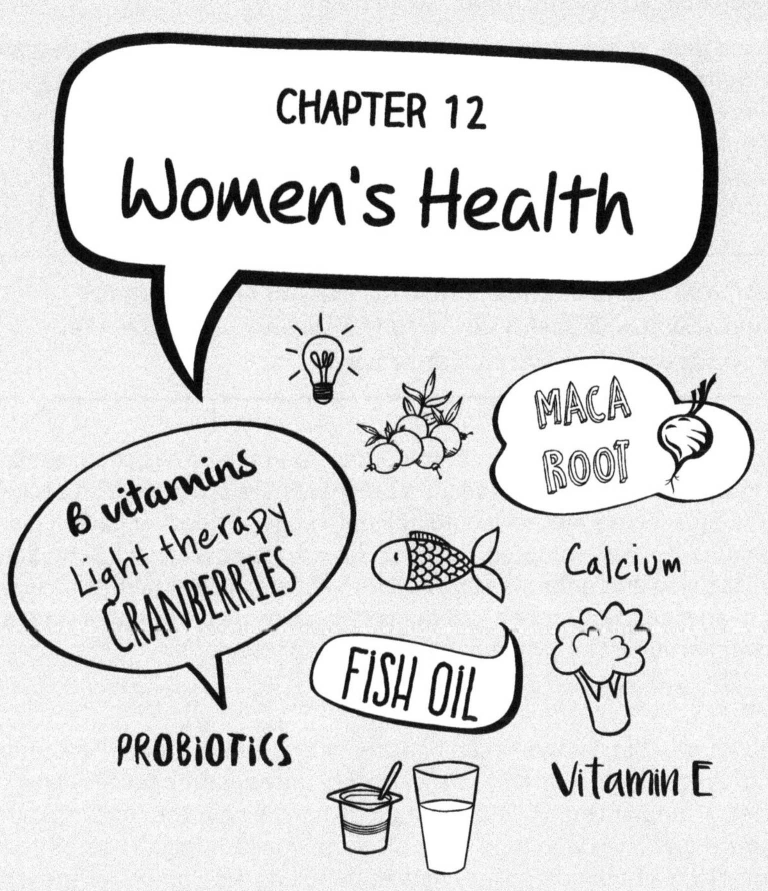

Life expectancy is higher for women than men in most countries. Despite this, they have their own personal set of health issues to deal with. Pregnancy, PMS and menopause are some of the health issues looked at in this chapter with natural remedies to help you handle them.

At any one time, about 5% of all women in the world are pregnant. Pregnancy can do weird things to your body. Many women experience food cravings while they are pregnant and 30% will crave something that is not edible during this time. Growing a new life can put a real strain on your body. By the second month of pregnancy, the amount of blood in the mother's body will have increased by 50%.

*It's not in all species of animals that the females are in charge of growing a baby; male seahorses carry their unborn young around in their bodies until they are ready to be born.*

Luckily the female body is much better understood than it has been in the past and ways to find out if a woman is pregnant have progressed. In ancient Egypt the prospective mother would pee onto bags of wheat or barley and if a certain type of grain sprouted, it meant she was going to have a baby. Later in 1927 the woman's urine was injected into female mice or rabbits to see if their ovaries reacted. Since 1978 the test can now be done with a simple home pregnancy test kit (without any mice being involved).

## Fish Oil

It is well known that omega-3s can boost your brainpower, but did you know that you can give your kids a head start before they are even born? Taking an omega-3 supplement while you are pregnant can help your baby's brain development. Women who took a fish oil supplement during the second and third trimesters of their pregnancy helped their kids develop better speech, were better behaved and had improved hand-eye coordination by the age of two.

Fish is, unsurprisingly, a good source of fish oil. Oily fish like salmon and mackerel contain more than white fish. Seeds and nuts also have high levels of omega-3 and can be a great vegetarian alternative.

*A good dose of fish oil supplement each day is 1000mg which should get you approx. 500mg of Omega-3.*

## B Vitamins

One lesser known symptom of pregnancy is painful leg cramps. Nearly 50% of pregnant women will experience them and they often occur at night during the final stages of pregnancy. No one is quite sure what causes these painful contractions of the calf muscles, but dehydration and fatigue have both been suggested as culprits.

Taking vitamins B1 and B6 has been shown to decrease your chances of getting leg cramps. A study showed that nearly three-quarters of pregnant women who had previously suffered from leg cramps experienced no leg pain when they took a vitamin B supplement.

Taking vitamin B supplements can also lower an older woman's risk of age-related macular degeneration (AMD), one of the leading causes of blindness in elderly people. A study of over 5,000 women showed you were a third less likely to suffer from AMD if you took vitamin B regularly.

## Light Therapy

Between 5% and 25% of new mothers are affected by postpartum depression after giving birth. Many have never experienced depression before in their life and may not believe or accept the diagnosis. It's normal to be worried about how medications may affect you when there are already so many things for you to think about and so some women will often not take antidepressants.

Light therapy may be the answer if you feel this way. Its benefits for seasonal affective disorder are well known and in a six week study light therapy improved depression symptoms in new mothers who had the treatment.

*In terms of getting exposure to light, outdoors on a sunny day is 50-100 times brighter than office or room lighting. Being outside on a cloudy day still gives a decent amount of light exposure.*

Light therapy involves exposing yourself to more light, typically using a light box although sunshine can be just as effective. Try to make your exposure earlier in the day to fit in with your body's natural rhythms and also so you can feel the benefits all day long.

## Vitamin E

Vitamin E was discovered in 1922 by Dr. Herbert Evans and Katherine Bishop. It wasn't until 1945, that scientists figured out that it was a great antioxidant. It protects your body from damage by free radicals, chemicals that roam the body stealing electrons from atoms and generally causing damage.

Taking vitamin E might be a good choice if you suffer from menopausal hot flushes. A study showed that taking vitamin E decreased the number of flushes from five to three each day in the participants and lowered the severity by 25%.

There is lots of food that you can get your vitamin E from with sunflower seeds, nuts and soybeans a being great place to start. If you are after something more exotic, give mango a try when they come into season.

## Maca Root

Grown high in the Andes mountains in Peru, the maca plant is related to the radish and the turnip. Like these vegetables, most of the plant is underground with only a few low-lying leaves visible from above. The root can be gold, cream, red, purple, blue, black, or green.

It has been long recognised in Peru for its ability to calm menopausal symptoms. It has been shown to reduce hot flushes, night sweats, anxiety, depression and heart palpitations. A study showed that 87% of women taking a maca root extract experienced lower levels of symptoms than women who did not.

*Hot flushes, also known as hot flashes in some part so the world, are a sudden feeling of warmth that begins in the face and chest and then spreads in waves to the rest of the body. It may not sound like much but it can be very uncomfortable.*

Maca root can be taken as an oral supplement and most Maca is grown high up the Andes mountains in Peru.

## Cranberries

These plump little red berries grow on a vine. They are white when they first appear and only turn red when they are ready to be eaten. A traditional accompaniment to Christmas dinners, they were first named *bearberries* due to the large appetite wild bears seemed to have for them.

Consuming cranberries on a regular basis can stop bacteria from attaching themselves to the walls of your bladder. A study showed that drinking cranberry juice reduced urinary tract infections, cystitis (inflammation of the bladder) and bladder stone formation.

Juice and sauce are just a few of the available forms of cranberry. They can also be eaten raw, dried, or sweetened. Cranberries can make an excellent alternative to blueberries in muffins or can add a different flavour to soups and stews. Cranberry supplements are also available; you will want around 400-800mg per day or 75ml of cranberry juice, but make sure it is pure juice.

### Black Cohosh

A flowering, white, woodland plant, black cohosh is native to North America. It has been used as a traditional remedy among Native Americans for sore throats, kidney pain and depression. Westerners have been using the herb to treat menopause since the 1700s. It contains vitamin C, selenium and many other nutrients that your body needs.

More importantly though, scientists think it may have an estrogen-like effect in your body. Many studies show that it can be effective at reducing the number of hot flushes you experience each day, in some cases halving them. It can also lower their intensity and reduce their length.

Black cohosh can be bought as a powder, fluid or tablet form, but do not take if pregnant.

*Warning: Black cohosh has many potential interactions with medicines that you may be taking, so this is a supplement that must be discussed with your doctor or pharmacist.*

### Soy

Only 25% of Japanese women experience hot flushes during menopause, compared to 85% of American women. There is a good theory that this might be due to the large amount of soy consumed daily in Asia. Substances in soy called *isoflavones* mimic estrogen in the female body. They plug into the estrogen receptors and trick your body into thinking there is more estrogen than you are actually producing.

Studies have shown this trickery to be very effective at reducing the number of hot flushes menopausal women experience each day.

There are some easy substitutions that you can make to increase the amount of soy in your diet. Choosing soy milk over dairy, or buying some roasted soy beans for snacking on are great ways to get more soy *isoflavones* into your body. Tofu and other meat alternatives are often soy based and can be made into main meals containing lots of soy.

### Chasteberry

It was once taken by monks to help them adhere more easily to their vows, which is why it earned itself the name *chasteberry*. Native to the

Mediterranean area, the first record of its use for medical purposes was by Hippocrates in Ancient Greece. He prescribed it for menstrual difficulties, and he might well have been onto something.

It's not well understood how chasteberry works but studies show that it can help to reduce symptoms of PMS. In one study of over 1,600 women, 93% reported that taking chasteberry either made their symptoms disappear completely or significantly improved them.

Chasteberry is unfortunately not a berry you can eat. Extracts of it can be bought in fluid, capsule or tea forms.

*There are several other names that it goes by, including vitex, chaste tree, Abraham's balm, lilac chastetree and monk's pepper!*

## Calcium

The number of pregnancy complications that calcium can help you avoid is truly astounding. A study of 8,000 pregnant women showed that calcium could reduce the risk of pre-eclampsia, eclampsia, gestational high blood pressure, low birth weight, preterm delivery and neonatal death.

Making sure you get enough calcium during pregnancy is very important. If you feel like you aren't eating enough dairy products, then a calcium supplement might be something for you to consider.

Calcium levels in your body tend to drop off before you get your period. Studies show that taking a calcium supplement to raise these levels can lower the severity of PMS symptoms and even may help you stay symptom-free.

## Probiotics

Probiotics boost the number of good bacteria in your body. The bacteria help fight off nasty infections in a number of ways, including by producing acid. The infectious bacteria don't like acidic conditions, so they grow more slowly and are less likely to cause a problem.

Low levels of bacteria in your vagina can cause an infection. This is normally harmless and cures itself, but if it happens during pregnancy there is a higher risk of miscarriage or harm to the growing foetus. Studies show that taking probiotics when an infection like this occurs is an effective cure either alone or with antibiotics.

Probiotic supplements are the best way to get all the good bacteria you need.

# CHAPTER 13
# Children's Health

Probiotics

Sulphur
Multivitamins
TEA TREE OIL

HONEY

ZINC

FISH OIL

In the ever-changing world of a growing body, there is so much to keep track of. Your brain has so much developing to do, you can't always communicate properly to say what's wrong, schools and playgrounds are a hotbed of infections and then to top it all off your skin goes haywire!

Growing a brain is a tough job. You are born with all the brain cells that you will ever have and by the age of three over half of these will have been '*pruned off*' as they are deemed unnecessary. 60% of a baby's energy is spent working on their brains. Parents will be pleased to know that your child crying when you leave them, is actually an important part of brain development; it shows that long-term memory is starting to kick in.

Sometimes though, babies can cry for no apparent reason. This is called colic, and is diagnosed by the rule of 3. If your baby cries for more than three hours, for more than three days a week, for over three weeks, then it is colic. It affects one in five babies and may be caused by gas or overstimulation.

The dreaded nits can be caught when lice jump from the head of an infected child to a new home on your child's head. They spread fast and adult lice can lay three to four eggs each day. All those creatures sucking on your blood can make you feel lousy, and this is actually the origins of that word! A novel natural treatment for this is described below.

Just when you are clear of childhood illnesses, stress, hormones and genetics can all cause acne to kick in. The six different types of acne spots vary in severity from the common whitehead to the nasty nodule. The old wives tale of the toothpaste cure for acne has not been tested in any good studies (although in theory it should help), but this chapter will offer you solutions to this and other problems.

## Sulphur

Sulphur occurs naturally all over the world, in volcanoes and underground eruptions. People have known about sulphur for many, many years. It is referenced in the bible under one of its past names, brimstone. Hell is said to smell of it. The phrase 'fire-and-brimstone' comes from this belief and means a sermon reminding you of the eternal damnation you may face.

*It's purely coincidence of course, but the rotten eggs smell that we all experience in Rotorua is from sulphur which is why it is sometimes nick-named the Sulphur City.*

Many acne products contain sulphur. Laboratory studies have shown that it can reduce the number of bacteria living on your face and clear up your acne.

Check the labels on different acne products to see if they contain any sulphur. Ideally you want to strike a balance between enough sulphur to clear up your face but not enough to leave you smelling of rotten eggs!

## Tea Tree Oil

Extracted (unsurprisingly) from the tea tree, this oil has been used by Aborigines for hundreds of years. The tea tree got its name when explorer Captain Cook attempted to boil its leaves to make a nice cup of tea. Its medical uses have definitely overtaken its beverage use, with tea tree oil being used to treat lice, wounds, burns and even toothache.

*Leptospermum scoparium is commonly called Mānuka, New Zealand tea tree or just tea tree; it is a species of flowering plant in the myrtle family Myrtaceae, native to New Zealand and to southeast Australia.*

Tea tree oil might also help reduce your acne. A study of over 120 young people showed that after 3 months tea tree oil reduced outbreaks and had fewer side effects than commonly used chemicals.

Tea tree oil (or Mānuka oil) can be applied as an ointment or cream. Soaps and lotions with tea tree oil extract in them can also be used.

## Zinc

Though its concentrations are highest in your bones, eyes, liver and pancreas, zinc is found in every cell in your body. Low levels of zinc have been associated with several different skin disorders.

Taking a zinc supplement might help reduce your acne. Studies show that zinc can decrease the numbers of pimples on your skin and in one study it was shown to be as effective as a commonly used acne drug.

You can get more zinc through your diet by eating the right types of food. Yoghurt, pecans and cashews are great, easy additions that will raise your zinc levels. Oysters, chicken thighs and pork tenderloins also contain lots of it. The mineral can also be taken as a supplement; for best results take on an empty stomach at night before bedtime.

## Hot Air

Using a hair dryer can be effective for more than just drying your hair. The heat can also be effective at ridding your scalp of lice and their eggs. Hot air was shown to kill 100% of eggs and 80% of hatched lice when used for 30 minutes. A study of 169 children showed that all the kids who underwent the heat treatment were cured of head lice a week later.

Unlike the chemicals that are often used to cure a case of head lice, the hot air will have no negative effects on you or your child's scalp. Make sure that you thoroughly cover all the areas of their head so that you get them all on your first try.

*For the best chance of success, use high heat and high speed settings, but be careful not to cause injury by heating the area too much.*

## Probiotics

It's not only adults who can need a top up of good gut bacteria. Infants can also benefit from the boost to their digestive system. If your baby has colic, then you might want to consider probiotics as a remedy.

A study of infants with colic showed that taking probiotics reduced their average crying time to just 51 minutes each day, compared to over two hours for babies who didn't take probiotics.

It's suggested that both mother and baby start taking probiotics together, especially if you are breastfeeding. Start with low doses, perhaps those found in drinking yoghurts, before increasing the amount taken.

## Fish Oil

Fish oil contains two important omega-3 fatty acids, eicosapentaenoic acid (EPA) and docosahexaenoic acid (DHA). EPA works in the blood, preventing clots, swelling and pain. DHA works to build your nervous system, including your brain.

Taking fish oil during pregnancy is thought to increase your child's intelligence, social skills and ability to communicate. Over 11,000 pregnant women took part in a study that showed eating more than 340g of seafood a week improved the brain development of their child.

It is often recommended that pregnant women avoid seafood because of the risk of trace contaminants of mercury. The risks of this are being revised, and so long as you avoid types of fish that are known to be high in mercury, it is generally assumed you are not putting your baby at risk. Salmon is a great example of a low-mercury, high fish oil species. If you are still worried though, fish oil supplements are safe to take throughout pregnancy.

## Multivitamins

Multivitamins are constantly being advertised as being able to do anything from ward off dementia to improve your sports performance. It's hard to know what's true, but one tried-and-tested function of multivitamins is to boost children's brain function. A study showed that after three months, children who had taken multivitamins performed better on attention span and other brain function tests than those who did not.

There is very little risk associated with taking a good multivitamin. They contain a variety of minerals and vitamins that your body needs to supplement what you might be missing out on in your diet. Anything that is not used by your body just gets flushed out. They are particularly good for 'fussy eaters' who may have low-grade vitamin or mineral deficiencies.

## Honey

A spoonful of sugar may help the medicine go down, but wouldn't it be great if the sugar was the medicine? For children who cough during the night, this might be the case. Night-time coughing can keep not just the sufferer, but the rest of the house up long into the night.

A study of over 100 children showed that taking honey around 30 minutes before they went to bed coated the nerve endings in their throat and reduced coughing. The honey can be eaten plain or mixed in with a soothing drink.

> *The good news is that for treating a cough, you can use any honey that you have in the house, it does not have to be expensive medical-grade or Mānuka honey.*

Medical-grade (sterile) honey has also been shown to be effective at reducing acne. A study of 135 people showed that honey improved acne within 2 weeks in many participants, with further improvements over the following 10 weeks of the study. It can reduce the severity and number of pimples and even your confidence in yourself. Make sure you use the sterilised medical-grade honey though, as nasty bacteria in edible honey can have the opposite effect. In addition, impurities in non-sterile honey can cause allergic reactions.

## Yoga

The name Yoga means to join, or to unite. It is about bringing the different parts of your body together and making you feel connected with yourself and the world around you. It can strengthen your body, improve your balance as well as make you feel content and calm.

For children going through rehabilitation, Yoga might help them connect with their bodies again. A systematic review of many studies decided that on an individual basis, Yoga could benefit young people.

> *Yoga does more than burn calories and tone muscles. It's a total mind-body workout that combines strengthening and stretching poses with deep breathing and meditation or relaxation.*

However a well-trained Yoga therapist will help you choose a pace that is right for you.

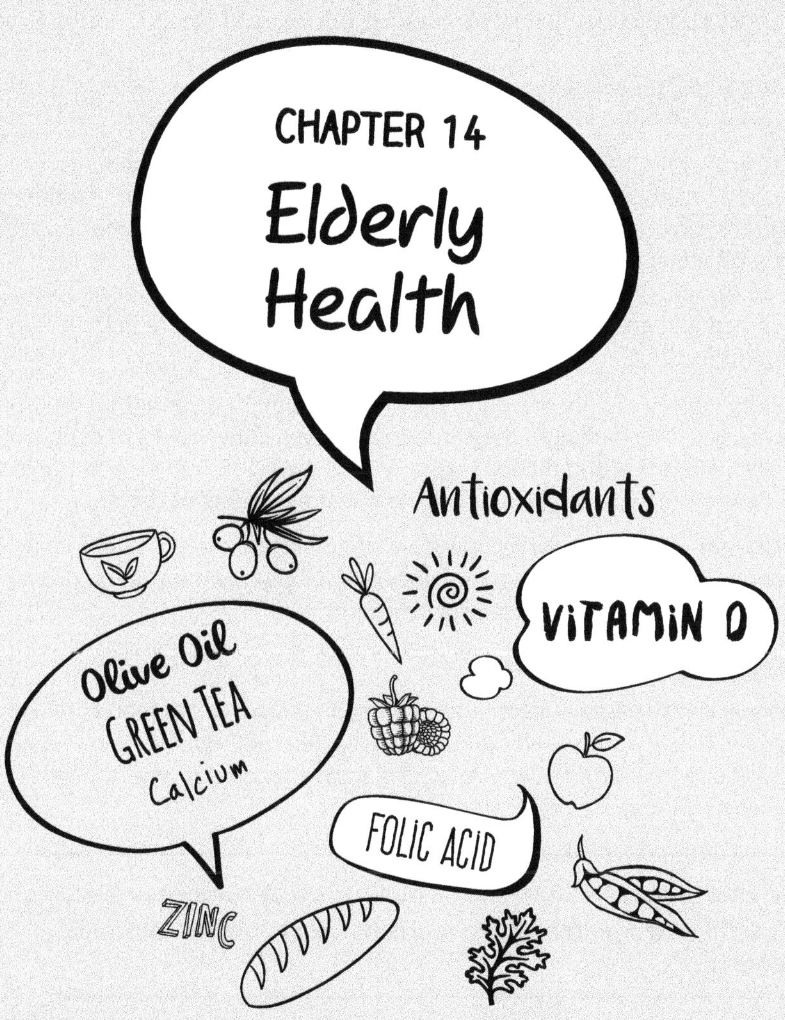
CHAPTER 14
Elderly
Health
Antioxidants
VITAMIN D
Olive Oil
GREEN TEA
Calcium
FOLIC ACID
ZINC

As life expectancy increases, so does the number of elderly people in society. It's estimated that there will be two billion people over the age of 60 by the year 2050 and they will make up over 20% of the world population. The number of elderly people may be growing, but you will actually shrink as you age. Your cells will start to collapse inwards and everything will become more concentrated. You also physically shrink by several inches as your spine gets worn away and more curved with the passing of the years.

Maybe one of the reasons your brain slows down as you grow older is because it has to search through so many years of knowledge to find the answer it's looking for. Tell that to your grand-children if they think you are being a bit slow! Wisdom and the ability to handle social situations are just two benefits that come with age and in many societies older people are revered and are the most important and respected people in their communities.

Brain and nerve cells are the only cells in your body that cannot be replaced and once they are damaged they are gone forever. Other types of cells, like skin cells, are lost and replaced regularly. You shed 600,000 skin cells every hour. By the time you are 80 you will have lost over 50kg of them!

This chapter will cover how to slow down some of the typical symptoms of aging, such as a decline in the quality of your sight, strengthening your bones, keeping safe from colds and infections.

## Antioxidants

When you get stressed, digest food, breathe in smoke or eat food with pesticides in them, your body releases nasty free radicals. Antioxidants work to stop these free radicals. Age-related macular degeneration is thought to be caused by these free radicals.

*Age-related macular degeneration (AMD) is a deterioration or breakdown of part of the eye, the macula, and is the most common cause of blindness.*

Increasing the number of antioxidants in your body can reduce your risk of AMD. A study of around 5,000 participants showed that antioxidants delayed the onset of AMD and reduced its symptoms. They might also slow down more advanced AMD, letting you keep your sight for longer.

Antioxidants are found in fresh fruit and vegetables. Making sure you get your 5+ a day is an important part of getting lots of antioxidants.

## Olive Oil

Olive oil can be tasted much like fine wine. You place a little in the glass and swirl it around to release the aromas. Good olive oil should smell like bananas, grass or apples. Bad olive oil might smell like cardboard, vinegar or mud. The natural polyphenols in olive oil might also be helpful at reducing age-related eye problems.

Heating olive oil destroys some of its flavour, but more importantly can also destroy some of the polyphenols that are meant to help you. Try using it as a salad dressing, or as a dip for your bread. This will let you enjoy the natural flavours of the oil as well as the health benefits of it.

## Zinc

Five million tonnes of zinc are mined each year by the world's leading zinc producer, China. In second place, Australia doesn't even manage half of that, mining only 1.5 million tonnes a year. Zinc is used in many metal alloys and coatings, but it might also help you stay infection free.

A study of healthy elderly people showed that taking a zinc supplement reduced the amount of infections they caught. This is probably due to the anti-inflammatory and antioxidant properties of zinc.

*Zinc deficiency symptoms include loss of appetite and an impaired immune function. In more severe cases, it can cause hair loss, diarrhoea and eye and skin lesions.*

Many multivitamins contain zinc. Natural food sources include whole-grain products, and seeds. Grainy brown bread might also be an excellent way to increase your zinc intake.

## Folic Acid

Folic acid, or vitamin B9, is important for making copies of your DNA. When your cells divide to make new cells, each cell needs a complete copy of your DNA in it, so folic acid is very important.

Low levels of folic acid might lead to poor hearing as your age. A study of over 7,000 elderly people showed that over a three year period, eating more folic acid was associated with better hearing.

Folic acid, or folate, is often added to food to help you get enough of this important vitamin. It is also present in leafy green vegetables, fruit and dried beans or peas.

### Vitamin D

Vitamin D is a compound that dissolves in fat. Having plenty of vitamin D in your body helps you to absorb other important nutrients like magnesium, calcium and iron.

Getting enough vitamin D might also reduce your risk of falling and injuring yourself. A study of 124 nursing home residents showed that taking vitamin D resulted in less falls and less broken bones than would have occurred if they were not taking vitamin D.

If you don't get out in the sun much, it's likely that you don't have enough vitamin D. Most of the vitamin D in your body is made when you are exposed to sunlight. Some food, like oily fish, oils, egg yolks and some meat contain a fair amount of vitamin D. Taking a supplement can be an easy way to ensure you get plenty of vitamin D each day.

*Public Health England recently said that millions of Britons should consider taking vitamin D supplements as many do not get enough from food/sun and the same applies to us here in New Zealand.*

### Green Tea

The oldest plant-based drink known to man, green tea has been drunk for over 4,000 years. It is a common beverage in Japan, where drinking several cups with each meal is not uncommon.

Drinking green tea could be the secret to a long and enjoyable life. A study of more than 40,000 Japanese adults showed that drinking two or more cups of green tea each day can potentially extend your lifespan and it approximately halved the chance of developing dementia or heart disease in this study.

Green tea can be drunk as you would drink regular tea or coffee. A cup when you wake up, one with your morning snack and perhaps one with your other meals. It can be brought as fresh tea leaves for a more authentic preparation, in tea bags for a quick and easy cuppa or in capsules for a more potent extract.

### Calcium

For a metal, calcium is quite soft and reacts easily with both air and water. In water it makes bubbles of hydrogen and it reacts with oxygen to form a white substance called calcium oxide. It's very important inside your body and is part of building and maintaining your bones.

Not having enough calcium in your body can increase your risk of breaking a bone and cause you to lose bone mass more quickly than you otherwise would. An analysis of 29 trials showed that elderly people reduced their breakages by 12% when they took a calcium supplement.

Dairy products are the obvious choice for calcium, but did you know that leafy green vegetables also include large amounts of it? If you are at high risk of breaking a bone, a calcium supplement might be the best choice for you.

*3% of the earth's crust is calcium. In humans, 99% of the calcium in our bodies is stored in the bones and teeth.*

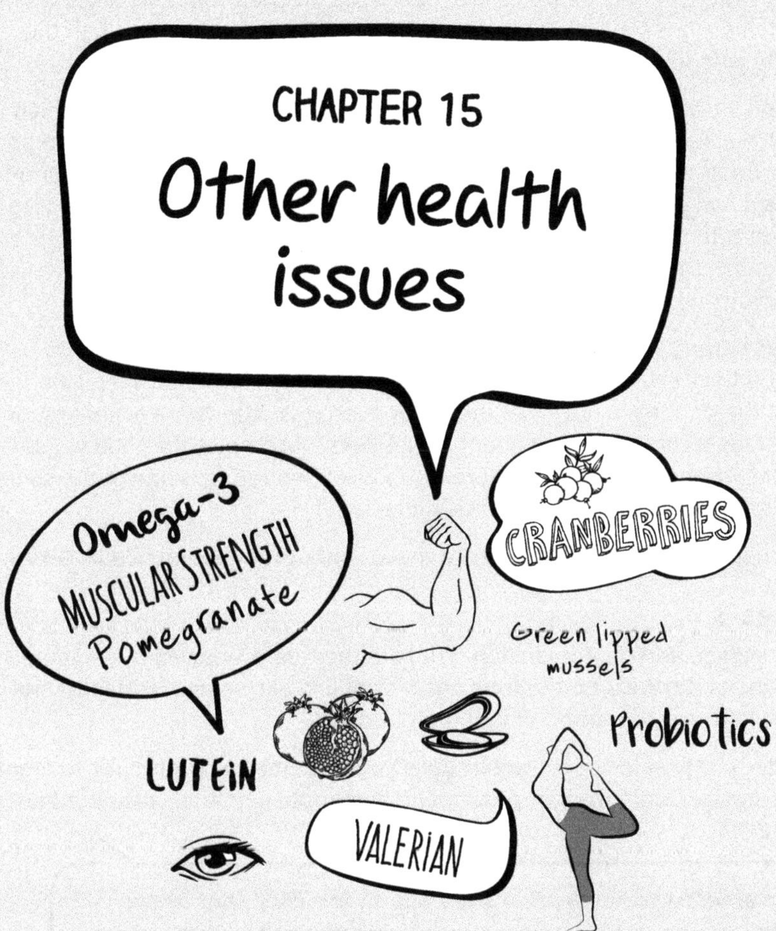
CHAPTER 15
Other health issues
Omega-3
MUSCULAR STRENGTH
Pomegranate
CRANBERRIES
Green lipped mussels
Probiotics
LUTEIN
VALERIAN

Around one third of adults will be affected by an allergy. Often, your immune system is labelling something that's actually harmless as a threat to your body. It goes into fight mode to try and get rid of the invading substance. One type of allergy is eczema. This is a recurring skin condition that causes rashes and itching. It is typically seen as a childhood illness, but around half the people who had it as a child will get it again as an adult.

It's well known that getting pregnant gets harder as you get older. Woman under the age of 35 shouldn't assume anything is wrong until you have been trying for at least a year, but once you reach the age of 35 that time period jumps down to six months. For a long time, men's age has been thought to be irrelevant to their fertility. New research is showing however, that the older your dad is the more likely you are to develop a mental health problem like autism or schizophrenia.

Humans aren't the only ones who suffer from insomnia. A study of flies showed that it was possible to select flies that slept less than average and breed them to make new flies that slept even less. After several generations, some flies slept less than an hour a day! These insomniac flies had worse balance, were fatter and had more trouble concentrating; some of the same symptoms as we see in human insomniacs.

This chapter offers you remedies to these, and other, general health issues.

## Omega-3

Marine algae and phytoplankton (krill) are the true producers of omega-3. From them, it travels up the food chain until fish like salmon and mackerel have a high concentration of it in their bodies.

Omega-3 fatty acids might well reduce your eczema symptoms. A two month study showed significant improvements in people who took a supplement of omega-3.

*This effect and many others, are due to the fact that omega-3 fatty acids reduce inflammation, which is the underlying problem in many diseases. In eczema, the skin gets inflamed.*

Supplements are one way to go, but omega-3 can also be obtained from the food you eat. Oily fish have lots of it in their bodies and it's recommended that you eat a portion of fish two to four times a week. Vegetarian sources are also available, try adding some flaxseed or chia to your diet.

## Pomegranate

For many millennia, the pomegranate has been linked with new birth and eternal life. In the past, this has been because of the hundreds of seeds it contains. In modern times, scientists have discovered the pomegranate may improve sperm quality and make men more fertile.

Studies showed that pomegranate extract increased the number of sperm and made them better swimmers.

Fresh pomegranate can be eaten by itself (a potentially messy venture) or the delicious insides can be added to many desserts, cakes or even cocktails. Pomegranate juice is an easy way for you to get ample amounts of the superfruit each day. Supplements with pomegranate extract are also an option, but make sure they include the beneficial seed, not just the flesh or juice of the fruit.

## Muscular Strength

Bulking up is often associated with gym nuts and fitness fanatics, but the science says it could benefit us all. The stronger you are, the longer you are likely to live.

A study of almost 9,000 men showed that being in the top third, strength-wise, reduced the likelihood of dying from all causes. This still held true when general overall fitness was accounted for.

The best way to grow muscle is resistance training. You should try to involve all of your major muscle groups and aim to give them a work out two or three times a week. Exercise equipment like rowing machines or weight machines can be a good way to achieve this, but more simple approaches like resistance bands or hand-held weights can also have great effects.

*Be wary of fad diets that often accompany strength training programmes and make sure you get all the nutrients you need or discuss with a nutrionist.*

## Cranberries

Cranberries grow on evergreen vines and blossom with pink flowers. It was these flowers that earned the fruit its name, as early American settlers thought they resembled the crane bird. The name *craneberry* became cranberry over time.

The main bacteria that causes dental decay is called *Streptococcus mutans* and cranberry can stop these bacteria in its tracks. Studies have shown that it can help fight tooth decay.

*Tooth decay, also known as cavities, or caries, is a breakdown of teeth due to activities of bacteria. The cavities may be a number of different colours from yellow to black. Symptoms may include pain and difficulty eating.*

Frozen, dried or fresh are just a few ways that cranberries can be enjoyed. Cranberry juice is a popular drink and a Christmas dinner would not be complete without cranberry sauce. Stopping tooth decay is one case where swallowing cranberry capsules are probably not helpful, as the cranberry needs to be in your mouth to work.

### Green lipped mussels

The New Zealand green-lipped mussel (or *Perna canaliculus*) lives all around the New Zealand coast. It is found mainly below the low-tide mark and it has been an important industry for the New Zealand economy for years. These special mussels contain certain types of omega-3 fatty acids and have anti-inflammatory properties that can benefit your whole body's health.

It has been shown to help with allergic conditions such as asthma, with joint conditions like arthritis and perhaps even slow mental decline in diseases such as Alzheimer's.

*Unfortunately, despite many media stories over the years, green-lipped mussel extract does not cure cancer. There were once some interesting studies done in test tubes, but it has not been shown to help cancer in humans.*

While a popular choice of seafood, it's not exactly to everyone's taste. If it's not your thing, don't worry freeze-dried powders and liquid capsules are also available for you to take.

### Beta-carotene

While you were probably told that carrots could help you see in the dark, there is very little evidence to support this. What you probably should have been told, is that carrots can stop you getting sunburnt! A substance in carrots known as beta-carotene should provide you with some sun protection and slow down the rate at which your skin burns. The larger the quantities you eat and the longer you keep your levels up, the better protection you get.

Carrots are obviously one good source of beta-carotene and it is this component which actually gives them their orange colour. Sweet potatoes and green leafy vegetables are other good options, or you might opt to take a supplement, which your body will convert to vitamin A as needed.

### Lutein

Its name comes from the Latin *luteus* meaning yellow and it is responsible for the bright yellow colour of egg yolks. It is important for helping the front parts of your eyes absorb blue light, protecting against damage that blue light causes to your retinas which are at the back of the eye.

Computer screens are often predominantly blue light, so lutein might help protect your eyes if you spend a lot of time looking at a computer screen. A study showed that after three months your eye's sensitivity to the contrast of a computer screen improved.

Egg yolks and green leafy vegetables are the top sources of lutein. In the study, the equivalent of a large spinach salads worth of lutein was eaten each day to get the best results. You can also buy supplements with lutein in them, which often include added zeaxanthin (a helpful addition for your eyes).

*Lutein is good for eyes in general. Other studies have found that it may reduce the chance of developing both age-related macular degeneration and cataracts.*

## Melatonin

Melatonin controls the day-night rhythm in humans and other animals. Basically, it guesses when you are going to want to sleep and gets your body ready in advance. Levels of melatonin go up when you are sleepy and down when you are awake. If you have insomnia, your melatonin levels could be the problem.

Taking a supplement of melatonin might help you get the sleep you desperately want. Studies have shown that melatonin increases 'sleep efficiency' meaning the ratio of time spent in bed to time spent asleep is much better.

The best way to take melatonin is as a supplement, a little while before you go to sleep. You may need to do a bit of experimenting to find the best dose and time for you.

*There are moves afoot to change the situation, but in New Zealand you currently need a prescription from a doctor to get melatonin. It is different in the USA where you can buy it from shops with no need for a prescription.*

## Valerian

Sweetly scented flowers bloom on the valerian plant in summer, but you wouldn't guess that by the scent of the extract, which is not that pleasant. It has been used as a herbal medicine since the time of ancient Romans and Greeks, and Galen was the first doctor to be recorded as using it to treat insomnia.

Taking valerian is still recommended if you have difficulty sleeping, particularly if this is due to stress. Several studies have shown that valerian can improve sleep and its potency is actually comparable to commonly prescribed insomnia drugs.

Valerian can be taken as a capsule, tablet or drunk as a tea. It's best to take it a little while before you go to bed, so it has time to start working before you try to sleep.

## Yoga

All exercise can make you more tired, so it makes a lot of sense that an exercise that includes relaxation and deep breathing might be a good way to help you sleep better at night. Yoga originated in India, but is now practiced all over the world. It incorporates poses, breathing and meditation and has all sorts of health benefits.

As yoga leaves you feeling calm and relaxed, it is no surprise that studies have shown that practicing Yoga just before bed can help you fall asleep more quickly.

There are lots of different types of Yoga. A gentle, calm style would definitely work best in this situation. Yoga classes can help you learn the basics so check out a community centre or gym to see if they are offered there, but best to leave your pyjamas at home.

## Pygeum

Prostate enlargement, technically known as benign prostatic hyperplasia (BPH), is when you have abnormal growth of your prostate that isn't related to an infection or tumour. No one is sure what causes it but it affects a large number of men. If you are over the age of 60, you have a 50% chance of having BPH!

Pygeum (African Plum Extract) is a plant extract that can relieve your symptoms. Studies have shown that it can reduce the number of times you need to go to the loo during the night and increase the effectiveness of each toilet break.

You won't want to eat the bark of the African plum tree so a supplement is your best option, expect to take around 75 to 200mg per day of the extract. Side effects are mild but can include nausea and stomach aches.

## Probiotics

These good bacteria still have a few benefits that haven't been mentioned yet. They can boost your immune system by stopping it from over-reacting to harmless substances and therefore reduce allergic reactions.

Studies showed that they could reduce the severity of hay fever symptoms and reduce your chance of developing eczema by around 18%. It does this by lowering the amount of the hormone that releases histamine and increasing the levels of the hormone that protects you from allergic reactions.

Tooth decay and bad breath are often caused by having too many bad bacteria in your mouth. Taking an edible or chewable probiotic supplement can slow down tooth decay and improve your breath by replacing the bad bacteria with good ones.

CHAPTER 16

# Staying safe with natural therapies

To finish this book we need to briefly talk about safety. It is widely and wrongly assumed that natural therapies are safe... because they are natural. This is simply not the case; cyanide is natural!

If any therapy affects the body and has a positive effect, it is also possible that it can also have a negative effect. Don't forget that around half of the medicines that a doctor can prescribe have their origins, directly or indirectly, in the natural world and as we all know, medicines can have side effects, sometimes nasty ones.

Another 'fact' that is widely and wrongly assumed is: if a low dose of a natural therapy is good for you, then a really big dose must be really really good for you! This is hardly ever the case and most times a really big dose will not have any extra benefit and may even be harmful.

A good example of this is vitamin C. We all need vitamin C and a small or moderate supplement can be great for our health. Some people however take this to the extreme and have infusions of massive doses of vitamin C directly into their veins. The doses that are used are often equivalent to the vitamin C that you would get from 700 oranges. This, not surprisingly, can be harmful.

There are many other extremes in the natural therapies world, another example being extreme diets which miss out whole food groups. Again, these are not recommended by most doctors or nutritionists. We need need a balanced diet, not an extreme one.

There is a range in the level of safety across the different types of natural therapies. Mind and body therapies such as meditation and yoga are considered to be safe on the whole, apart from maybe the odd pulled muscle. But when it comes to herbal medicines for example, some of these can be very potent and so there is more risk of harm. As well as having side effects that can be detrimental to health, they can also potentially interact with prescribed medications that you may be taking.

These 'drug-herb' interactions can be in one of two directions: the herbs can potentially increase the potency of the prescribed medicine, and you can suffer side effects as a result. Also it is often forgotten that the herbs can reduce the effectiveness of the prescribed medication and this can be catastrophic when taking important medicines such as antibiotics for bacterial infections or chemotherapy for cancer.

Another area of concern is product quality of natural products and there are two issues here. Firstly, does the product contain the ingredients that it says on the label and have the correct amount? There have been many examples where consumers have been ripped off from products delivering only a fraction of the dose that it should, omega-3 fish oil supplements being a frequent culprit.

Secondly, there have also been many examples of products being contaminated, such as high levels of lead being found in some supplements imported from overseas and high levels of mercury in fish oil supplements. What can you do about this?

The best option you have is simply to shop from a reputable company and choose a reputable brand. Yes, you may pay a bit more, but it's a good investment as these companies and brands invest time and money into ensuring the quality of their products.

There is one more important area in which the use of natural therapies and products can be harmful. It cannot be emphasized enough that you should use natural therapies **with** and not instead of other treatments that your doctor or other healthcare professional recommend for you. Ideally your doctor will be involved in the decision about using the natural therapy as well.

We see lots of problems when people delay using good, proven, medical treatments because they want to try natural therapies first. Sometimes, the delay in using the proven medical treatment can be harmful, or even fatal. Worst still, some people choose not to use standard medical treatments at all and choose to use just natural therapies. In other words they are using them as *alternative* therapies rather than *complementary* therapies. This very rarely ends well.

Finally, it cannot be stressed enough that this book is a very brief overview of dozens of natural therapies and so it should not be taken as an instruction manual for your health. Instead, please use it as a starting point to get more information on a therapy or therapies that you might want to try.

It's a cliché but still very important: healthcare decisions, including which natural therapies to take should be discussed with a qualified doctor or other healthcare professional such as a pharmacist. Pharmacists tend to be more up-to-speed with natural products but an increasing number of doctors are learning about them and recommending them as useful additions to standard treatments.

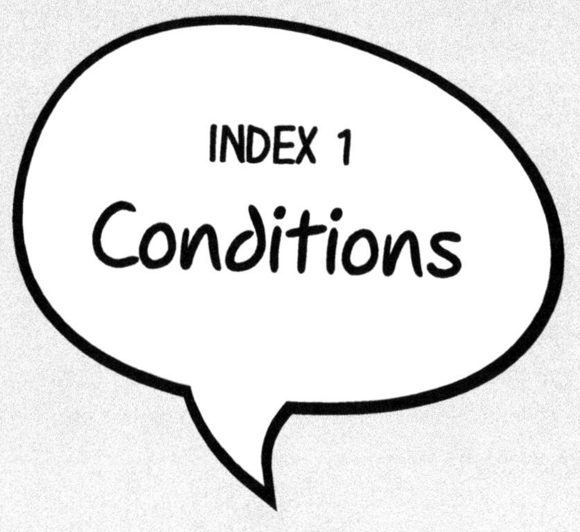
INDEX 1
Conditions

# Conditions


Aches 10, 18, 118
AIDS 58, 90
Alert 14
Allergy 37, 114
Alzheimer's disease 62, 63, 64, 67, 116
Anxiety 55, 65, 67, 72, 73, 74, 75, 76, 80, 98
Arrhythmias 48
Arthritis 10, 82, 86, 87, 88, 116
Attention deficit / hyperactivity disorder (ADHD) 62, 66, 67
Autistic 66
Autoimmune 27, 32, 60, 63, 82, 87
Back pain 4, 18
Bipolar Disorder 80
Bladder Stone 98
Bloating 55, 58, 60
Blood 10, 12, 21, 27, 34, 35, 36, 37, 38, 39, 42, 43, 44, 45, 46, 47, 48, 49, 50, 52, 54, 64, 67, 68, 69, 73, 75, 77, 78, 79, 80, 83, 85, 86, 90, 96, 100, 102, 104
Blood Clots 43, 48
Blood Flow 42, 67, 86
Blood Pressure 42, 43, 44, 45, 46, 47, 48, 50, 52, 73, 80, 85, 100
Blood Sugar 35, 36, 37, 38, 39, 54
BMI 11
Bones 10, 22, 27, 29, 36, 40, 65, 82, 83, 84, 85, 88, 92, 103, 108, 110, 111
Bowel Cancer 94
Bowels 55, 58, 60
Brain 18, 32, 46, 58, 62, 63, 64, 66, 67, 68, 72, 73, 74, 75, 78, 90, 96, 102, 104, 105, 108
Breast 15, 87, 90, 103
Breast Cancer 90, 92, 93, 94
Breathing 18, 26, 29, 30, 31, 32, 65, 73, 76, 77, 106, 118
Burns 12, 19, 87, 103, 116
Cancer 3, 4, 5, 21, 36, 58, 86, 87, 90, 91, 92, 93, 94, 116, 122
Cartilage 82, 85, 88
Children's Health 101

Cholesterol 38, 39, 42, 43, 44, 45, 48, 49, 50, 51, 52
Cold 4, 26, 27, 28, 30
Colic 102, 104
Colorectal 90, 91, 92
Constipation 39, 56, 59, 60
Cough 105
Cramps 21, 46, 55, 56, 58, 97
Crohn's disease 37, 60
Cuts 12, 15
Cystitis 98
Dementia 62, 63
Dental decay 115
Depression 72, 73, 74, 75, 77, 78, 79, 80, 97, 98, 99
Diabetes 10, 34, 35, 36, 37, 38, 39, 40, 80, 94
Diarrhoea 4, 39, 54, 55, 57, 58, 59, 60, 109
Diet 2, 10, 11, 16, 28, 29, 31, 34, 36, 37, 40, 47, 48, 50, 52, 60, 62, 68, 83, 90, 91, 92, 99, 103, 105, 114, 122
Difficulty moving 82
Digestion 22, 38, 50, 54, 56, 93
Digestive 11, 28, 54, 55, 56, 58, 59, 60, 91, 92, 104
Digestive tract 54
Disease 10, 13, 23, 26, 27, 32, 35, 37, 38, 40, 42, 43, 44, 45, 47, 48, 49, 52, 60, 62, 63, 66, 67, 78, 79, 82, 87, 90, 94, 110
Dizziness 44, 46, 80
Drowsiness 44
Dying 26, 48, 90, 115
Dysmenorrhea 21
Eczema 114, 119
Elderly Health 107
Energy 10, 12, 13, 28, 34, 38, 45, 48, 50, 54, 69, 83, 94, 102
Epilepsy 62, 64
Exercise 2, 3, 10, 12, 13, 14, 15, 28, 30, 45, 48, 55, 59, 63, 66, 74, 78, 94, 118
Eyes 15, 20, 34, 42, 69, 73, 103, 117
Fat 11, 12, 21, 31, 38, 42, 47, 49, 57, 90, 91, 110
Fatigue 23, 44, 80, 97
Fear of flying 57

## Conditions cont..

Fibromyalgia 4, 18, 20, 22, 23
General wellbeing 74
Giving up smoking 57
Hand-eye coordination 96
Headache 44, 45, 46, 65, 69, 70, 80
Head lice 104
Heal 12, 22, 77
Hearing 109
Heartburn 35, 55
Heart Disease 10, 13, 35, 37, 38, 42, 43, 44, 45, 47, 48, 49, 52, 94, 110
Helicobacter pylori infection 60
Hormones 22, 72, 77, 80, 84, 102
Hot flushes 98, 99
Hydration 13
Immune 26, 27, 28, 29, 31, 32, 57, 67, 75, 80, 82, 84, 109, 114, 118
Indigestion 55, 87
Infections 4, 12, 26, 27, 30, 39, 55, 60, 98, 100, 102, 108, 109, 122
Inflammation 31, 54, 87, 98, 114
Inflammatory Bowel 60
Injury 14, 15, 63, 74, 104
Insomnia 45, 76, 114, 117, 118
Intestines 16, 38, 39, 50, 54, 56, 58
Irritable bowel syndrome (IBS) 55, 56, 59, 60
Kidney pain 99
Lifespan 110
Ligaments 18, 65, 66
Listening skills 62
Lung Cancer 86, 90, 94
Lungs 12, 46
Macular Degeneration 97, 108, 117
Memory 23, 36, 45, 62, 63, 64, 85, 102
Menopause 10, 96, 99

Mental illnesses 72, 73
Migraines 62, 65, 66, 68, 69
Mood 18, 22, 23, 47, 69, 72, 75, 77, 79, 80
Morning sickness 55
Multiple sclerosis 32, 62, 63
Muscle 14, 15, 29, 46, 50, 57, 66, 68, 115, 122
Nausea 4, 30, 44, 45, 54, 55, 57, 58, 59, 65, 69, 70, 76, 118
Nervous system 34, 61, 63, 64, 104
Night sweats 98
Nutrients 11, 16, 22, 47, 49, 50, 54, 56, 57, 58, 63, 64, 79, 91, 93, 99, 110, 115
Osteoarthritis 19, 82, 85, 86, 87
Osteoporosis 83
Outlook 20
Pain 4, 14, 15, 18, 19, 20, 21, 22, 23, 46, 50, 54, 59, 60, 66, 68, 69, 75, 80, 82, 85, 86, 87, 88, 97, 99, 104, 115
Palpitations 98
Pancreas 21, 22, 54, 103
Pancreatitis 54
Period pain 21
PMS 96, 100
Pregnancy 38, 73, 96, 97, 100, 104
Prostate 118
Recovery 14
Relaxation 2, 45, 47, 65, 73, 85, 106, 118
Rheumatoid arthritis 82, 86, 87, 88
Rickets 27
Scar 15
Schizophrenia 80, 114
Sight 65, 108
Sleep 23, 32, 59, 65, 78, 117, 118
Sore mouth 69
Sore throats 26, 99
Spasms 66, 68
Speech 96
Sperm 115
Sprain 15

## Conditions cont..

Stiffness 82, 85, 86, 88
Stomach 16, 22, 29, 30, 44, 54, 55, 56, 58, 60, 80, 103, 118
Strains 18, 60, 96
Stress 45, 47, 59, 65, 67, 72, 76, 77, 80, 102, 118
Stroke 48, 49, 50, 94
Sunburn 21
Sweating 19, 44
Swelling 15, 31, 43, 54, 56, 68, 82, 85, 86, 88, 104
Teeth 12, 40, 48, 83, 111, 115
Tendons 18, 66
Ulcerative colitis 60
Ulcers 37, 60
Urinary tract infections 98
Virus 58
Vomiting 30, 54, 55, 57, 58, 59, 60
Weight 6, 10, 11, 12, 13, 16, 48, 60, 62, 100, 115
Women's Health 95
Workouts 10, 13, 30, 106
Wounds 15, 87, 90, 103

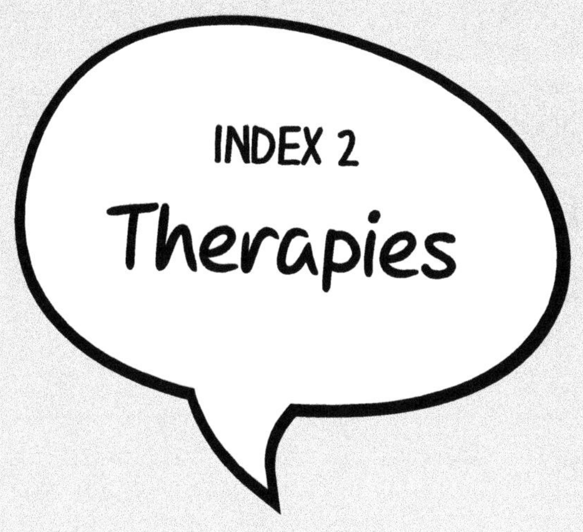
INDEX 2
Therapies

# Therapies


5-HTP **75, 76**
Alcohol **48, 49, 75, 76**
Alpha-Lipoic Acid (ALA) **38**
Amino acids **12**
Antioxidants **22, 31, 32, 43, 65, 91, 108**
Aromatherapy **2, 3, 74**
Art Therapy **77**
Asthma **26, 27, 29, 30, 31, 37, 116**
Avocado **91**
Baths **19, 22, 86**
Berries **22, 43, 65, 98**
Beta-carotene **116**
Biofeedback **73**
Black Cohosh **99**
Boswellia Serrata **85**
Breathing **18, 26, 29, 30, 31, 32, 65, 73, 76, 77, 106, 118**
Butterbur **68**
B Vitamins **66, 78, 79, 83, 97**
Caffeine **10, 14, 30, 32, 75, 94**
Calcium **10, 11, 13, 36, 40, 42, 43, 49, 50, 83, 84, 92, 100, 110, 111**
Capsaicin **10**
Chasteberry **99, 100**
Chilli **15**
Chiropractic **3, 22, 23**
Chondroitin **85**
Chromium **38, 79**
Cinnamon **39**
Coenzyme Q10 **50, 69, 70**
Colostrum **57**
Compression Stockings **45**
Cranberries **64, 98, 116**
Dance and Movement Therapy **78**
Devil's Claw **87**

DHEA 84
Diet 2, 3, 10, 11, 16, 28, 29, 31, 34, 36, 37, 40, 47, 48, 50, 52, 60, 62, 68, 75, 83, 90, 91, 92, 99, 103, 105, 114, 122
Echinacea 27
Electrolytes 13
Exercise 2, 3, 10, 12, 13, 14, 15, 28, 30, 45, 48, 55, 59, 63, 66, 74, 78, 94, 118
Fenugreek 39
Feverfew 69
Fibre 34, 35, 40, 50, 51, 56, 59, 75, 93
Fish Oil 3, 13, 14, 19, 47, 48, 62, 80, 88, 91, 95, 96, 104, 123
Flavonoids 44
Folate 78, 83, 93, 94, 109
Fruit and vegetable juice 63
Garlic 35, 46, 47
Ginkgo Biloba 67
Ginseng 26, 37, 93
Glucosamine 19, 20, 88
Green lipped mussels 116
Green tea 10, 11, 12, 32, 47, 94, 110
Guar Gum 39, 40
Hawthorn 44
Heat Therapy 19
Honey 15, 34, 105
Hot Air 103, 104
Hypnosis 3, 57, 78
Ice 15, 91
Kava 76
Kiwifruit 29, 56, 67
L-arginine 12
Light Therapy 79, 97
L-ornithine 12, 13
Lutein 116, 117
Maca 98
Magnesium 13, 29, 36, 40, 48, 68, 84, 110
Massage 2, 3, 7, 65, 66, 72, 73, 85
Meditation 3, 7, 18, 45, 47, 66, 67, 73, 77, 106, 118, 122

## Therapies cont..

Melatonin 46, 117
Multivitamins 12, 105, 109
Muscular Strength 115
Music 3, 7, 20, 77, 78
Niacin 45, 83
Nuts 12, 28, 29, 31, 36, 40, 45, 48, 49, 52, 65, 66, 68, 96, 98, 115
Oats 51
Olive Oil 49, 66, 90, 91, 109
Omega-3 3, 13, 14, 31, 35, 47, 48, 62, 66, 80, 87, 88, 91, 96, 104, 114, 116, 123
Omega-6 66
Optimism 75
Osteopathy 3, 65
Osteotherapy 22, 23
Pancreatitis 54
Peppermint oil 55
Physiotherapy 14
Phytosterols 51
Pine Bark 21, 37, 46, 65
Plant Stanols 51
Pomegranate 114, 115
Prebiotics 11, 55, 56
Probiotics 16, 28, 29, 56, 58, 59, 60, 100, 104, 118
Psyllium 38, 50, 51, 56
Pycnogenol 21, 31, 32, 37, 46, 65, 85
Pygeum 118
Riboflavin 69, 83
R.I.C.E 15
SAMe 80
Seaweed 86, 87
Selenium 44, 45, 99
Soy 44, 51, 52, 82, 83, 99
Spa Therapy 86

Sports drinks **13**
St John's Wort **80**
Stress Management **47**
Sulphur **102, 103**
Synbiotics **56, 57**
Tai Chi **47, 73, 74, 87**
Tea Tree Oil **103**
Tryptophan **75**
Tyrosine **10**
Ultra Violet (UV) **20, 21**
Valerian **76, 117, 118**
Vitamin B2 **69**
vitamin B9 **83, 93, 109**
Vitamin C **30, 43, 46, 47, 84, 99, 122**
Vitamin D **16, 21, 27, 36, 40, 42, 43, 63, 74, 91, 92, 110**
Vitamin E **29, 46, 67, 68, 97, 98**
Vitamin K1 **36, 37**
Vitamin K2 **84**
Water **13, 19, 22, 35, 39, 40, 46, 50, 56, 59, 74, 82, 86, 87, 94, 110**
Yoga **3, 18, 19, 45, 47, 54, 55, 64, 65, 77, 105, 106, 118, 122**
Zinc **12, 28, 103, 109**

www.ingramcontent.com/pod-product-compliance
Ingram Content Group UK Ltd.
Pitfield, Milton Keynes, MK11 3LW, UK
UKHW020140250726
13967UKWH00002B/780